Laser / IPL Technology for Skin Care

A comprehensive technical and informative textbook

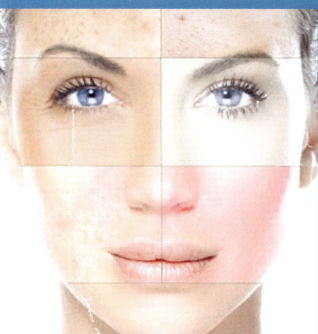

New Concepts & Techniques

For:

Practitioners
Students
Clinics
Public

1

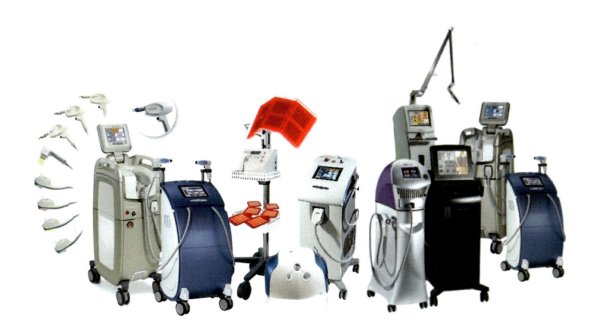

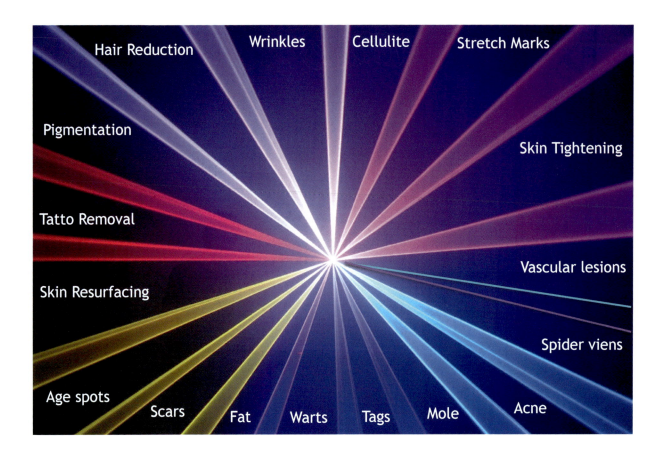

Author:

Dr. Dariush Honardoust

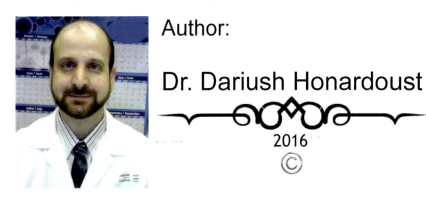

2016
©

President & director of the Canadian Association of Medical Spas & Aesthetic Surgeons
Doctorate: CranioFacial, Faculty of Dentistry, University of British Columbia, Canada
Postdoctorate: Division of Plastic Surgery, University of Alberta, Canada
Anatomy & Cell Biology, University of Western Ontario, Canada
Professor, BC Academy of Medical Aesthetics & Skin Care

Dr. Dariush Honardoust has earned his academic expertise in Canada including Doctorate: CranioFacial, Faculty of Dentistry, University of British Columbia, Postdoctorate: Division of Plastic Surgery, University of Alberta, and Master's degree in Anatomy & Cell Biology, University of Western Ontario. The highlights of his qualifications include excellent record of teaching and clinical and research productivity and manuscript publications, conducting research projects and training graduate and undergraduate students, student advising and curriculum development. Dr. Honardoust is the president of the Canadian Association of Medical Spas and Aesthetic Surgeons. He also serves as the teaching professor at the prestigious BC Academy of Medical Aesthetics & Skin Care.

Disclaimer:

Practitioners must always rely on their own experience and knowledge in evaluating and using any information, methods, compounds, or experiments described herein. In using such information or methods they should be mindful of their own safety and the safety of others, including parties, for whom they have a professional responsibility.

With respect to any drug or pharmaceutical products identified, readers are advised to check the most current information provided on procedures featured or by the manufacturers of each product to be administered, to verify the recommended dose or formula, the methods and duration of administration, and contradictions. It is the responsibility of practitioners, relying on their own experience, and knowledge of their patience, to make diagnosis, to determine dosages and the best treatment of each individual patient and to take all appropriate safety precautions.

To the fullest extent of the law, the author shall not assume any liability for any injury and / or damage to persons or property as a matter of products liability, negligence, or otherwise, or from any use or operation of any methods, products, instructions or ideas contained in the material herein.
January 2016

- Basic skin biology
- Anatomy and Physiology of Human Skin
- Basic hair biology and growth cycles
- Facial rejuvenation and skin resurfacing concepts by lasers
- Tattoo removal and pigmentation reduction
- Sanitation and disinfection methods
- Laser and IPL hair removal
- Physics of Lasers
- Laser safety
- Laser operating procedures on clients
- Contraindications & good candidates
- Equipment testing and maintenance
- Laser parameters (Wavelength, pulse duration, spot size, energy settings).
- Different types of cosmetic and medical lasers
- Lasing Mediums and Materials
- Laser safety for clients and practitioners
- Skin typing and proper selection of energy (fluence) level
- Pre- and post- laser assessment and treatment
- Client consultations
- Patient observation

Table of Contents

Definition...11
How laser light is generated?...21
Characteristic of laser light..26
Laser Mechanism of Action...34
Basic components of a laser emitting system................................45
Light interaction with tissue...57
Laser / IPL adjustment parameter...64
Wavelength, Fluence, Pulse Duration..66
Types of cosmetic and medical lasers..83
ND-YAG, Ruby, CO2, Erbium, Diod, Alexandrite, and IPL..............89
Safety for cosmetic laser procedures...130
Procedures that you can perform with a laser / IPL system............154
Skin Tightening..156
Skin Resurfacing (Ablative and non-ablative)...............................163
Hyperpigmentation Removal...174
Vascular Lesions / Spider Vein Removal......................................180
Tattoo Removal..186
Hair Reduction by Laser / IPL...195
Acne treatment..214
Preparation of clients prior to a laser treatment...........................220
Contraindications...233
Post-treatment care...244
Glossary...254

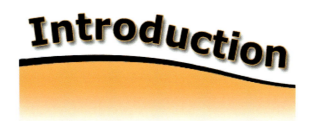

Introduction

This textbook provides a comprehensive overview of how lasers and IPL devices work including the physics of lasers / IPL. The most commonly used dermatologic lasers and their mechanism of action are discussed in the following chapters.

The topics include parameters used for effective cosmetic laser procedures, photo-facial, treatment of vascular and pigmented lesions, hair reduction, tattoo removal, and skin tightening and rejuvenation. Laser / IPL tissue interaction, acne treatment, skin typing, and operational safety measures are discussed in details. Discussion of the management and treatment of adverse side effects, the benefits, expected results and outcomes, and available alternative options are also presented. Focus on patient consultation, selection and education, safety and efficacy issues and important criteria for a successful treatment outcome in this textbook make it a very good source for quick reference.

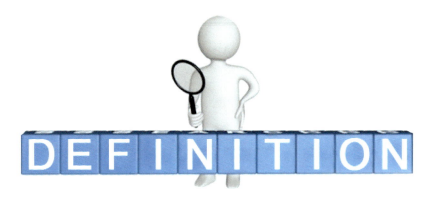

The word LASER stands for Light Amplification by the Stimulated Emission of Radiation. Laser therapy can be used to treat a variety of normal and pathological conditions. Several dermatology / cosmetic laser systems are available in the market for the treatment of various skin conditions such as hair removal, facial wrinkles, acne, acne and surgical scars, moles, melasma, stretch marks and sun damage.

Compared to other procedures such as chemical peels, cosmetic laser therapy has been found to be better tolerated by patients and cause less discomfort. The side effects are transient and include sensation like a prickly heat during treatment. In addition, a slight facial redness and swelling associated with laser treatment may occur that last for a few hours to days. Different types of lasers emit specific colors of light and are used to treat various skin conditions and problems. The laser light is generated by a monochromatic light emission sourced from a lasing medium. Depending on a specific wavelength, the monochromatic coherent and polarized beams of the light permit penetration into the skin in different depth. The photons of light energy that are absorbed by a variety of micro-molecules within the cells or tissues, initiates a number of physiological responses.

L.A.S.E.R

Definition

- **L**ight
- **A**mplification
- **S**timulation
- **E**mission
- **R**adiation.

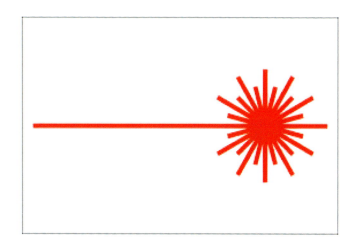

13

Laser / IPL is Non-ionizing radiation of light, like these forms of radiations:

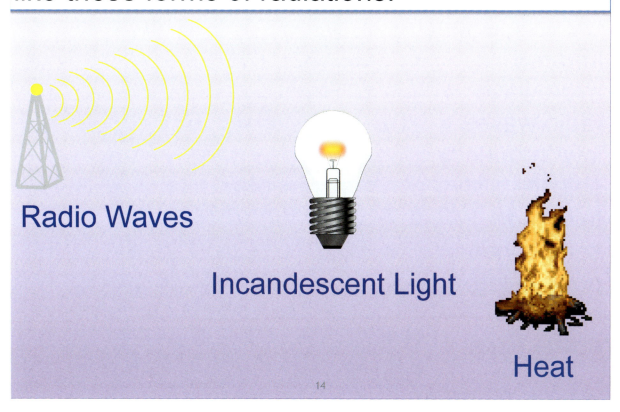

Radio Waves

Incandescent Light

Heat

14

Non-ionizing radiation:

Refers to any type of electromagnetic radiation that does not carry enough energy per quantum to ionize atoms or molecules.

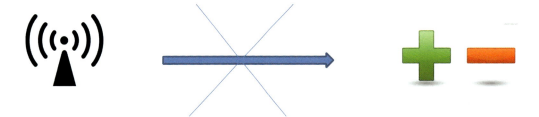

Non-ionizing radiation can produce non-mutagenic effects such as inciting thermal energy in biological tissue that can lead to structural changes. 15

Examples of non-ionizing radiation

UV visible light
infrared
microwave
radio waves
low-frequency
satellite dish
television
cell phones
power plug
computer
power lines

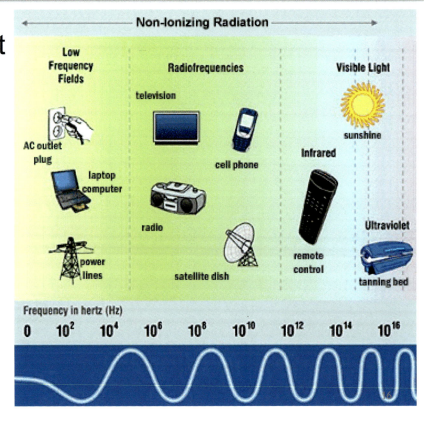

Ionizing radiation:

An Ionizing Radiation is composed of particles that individually carry enough kinetic energy to liberate an electron from an atom or molecule, ionizing it.

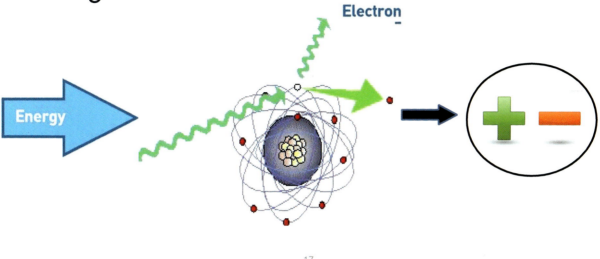

Ionizing radiation is generally harmful and potentially lethal to living things.

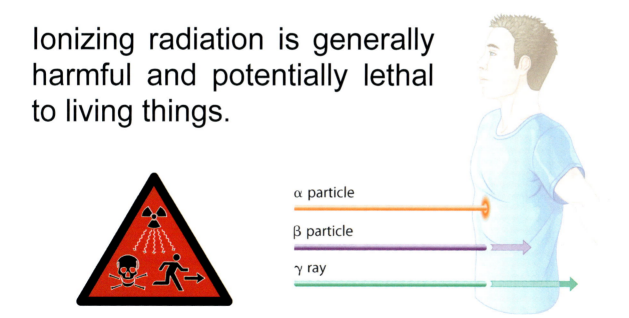

It is mutagenic leading to DNA mutation and cancer development. High doses can cause visually dramatic radiation burns, and/or rapid fatality through acute radiation syndrome.

Ionizing radiation can have curing benefits in radiation therapy for the treatment of tumours and thyrotoxicosis.

Controlled doses are used for medical imaging and radiotherapy.

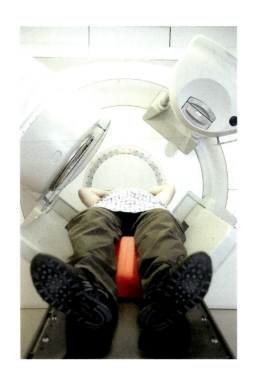

Examples of ionizing radiation

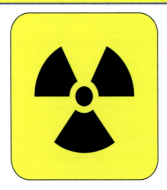

Nuclear radiation, along with gamma rays and x-rays are ionizing forms of radiation, meaning that exposure to them can cause cell mutation and/or death.

How Laser light is generated?

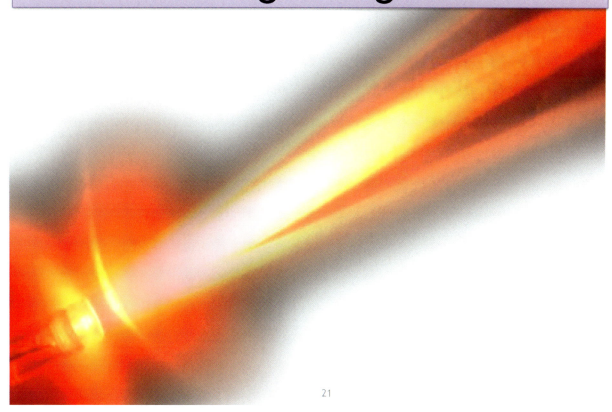

Electrons are usually in a "resting" stage; when they absorb a photon, they are raised to an "excited" stage.

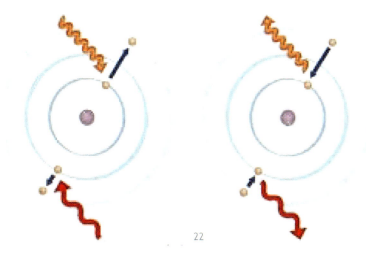

Once raised to an "excited" stage, the electron naturally tends to return to its "resting" stage, and does so by emitting a photon (similar to the one absorbed): this is called <u>spontaneous</u> <u>emission</u>.

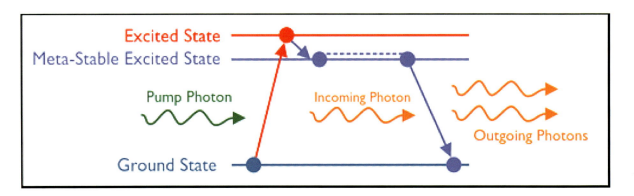

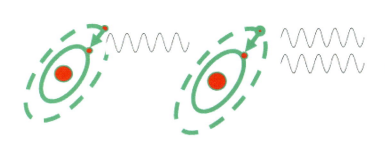
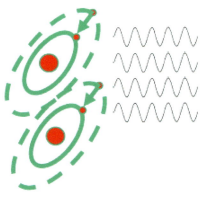

The laser atom spontaneously emits a photon (light)...

The photon stimulates another atom to emit a photon that is in-phase with the first photon and these photons...

...stimulate more atoms to emit light in-phase with the very first photons, etc...

The generated laser beam is a non-divergent strong coherent radiation

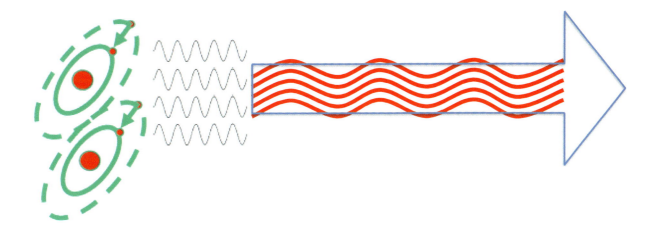

Characteristics of laser light

Characteristics of laser light: (1)

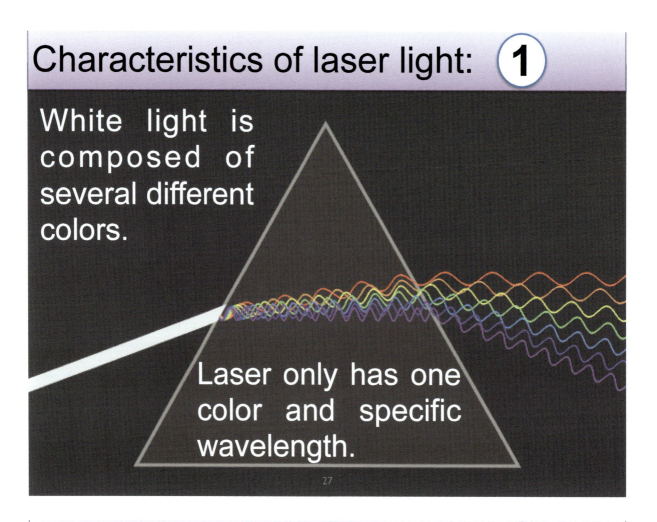

White light is composed of several different colors.

Laser only has one color and specific wavelength.

Characteristics of laser light: (2)

Laser light is Monochromatic.

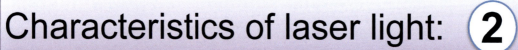

Regular white light is composed of different colors (Multichromatic).

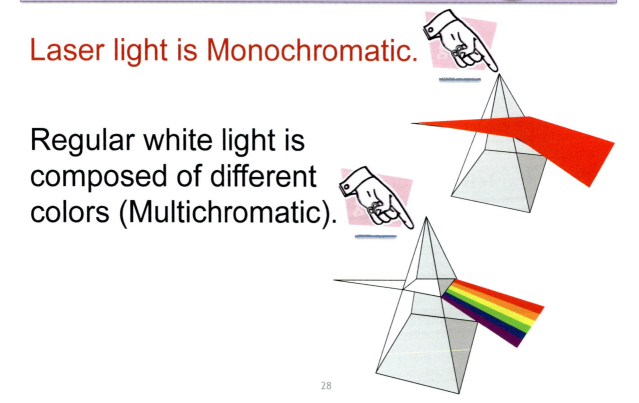

Wavelength: Each color has specific wavelength and frequency.

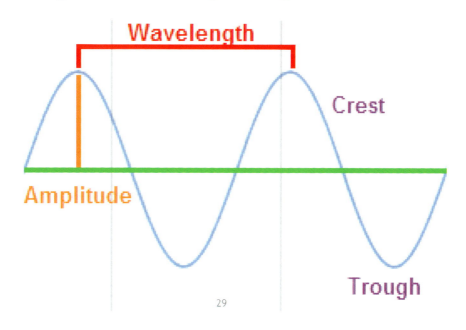

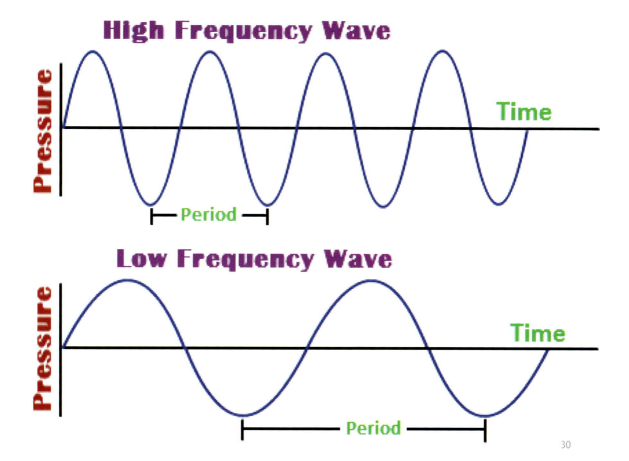

Characteristics of laser light: 4

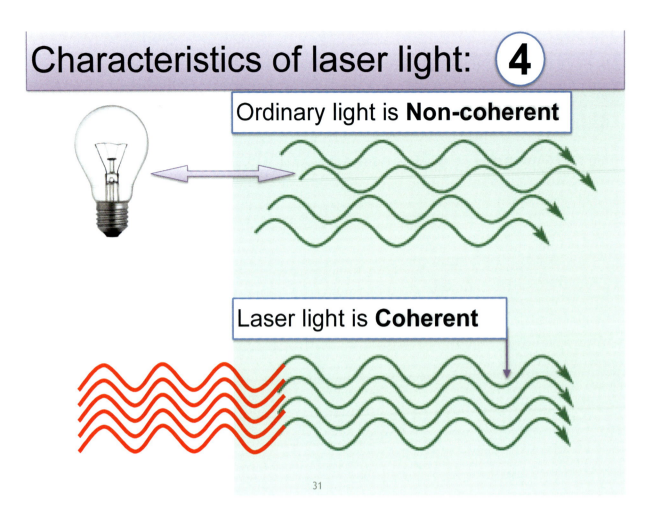

Ordinary light is **Non-coherent**

Laser light is **Coherent**

Characteristics of laser light: 5

Laser light is Collimated or (non-divergent).

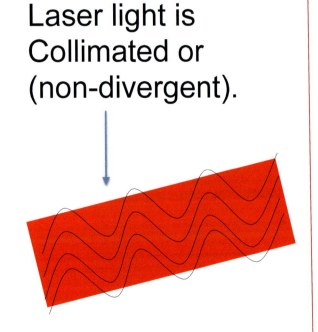

Ordinary light is Non-collimated or (divergent).

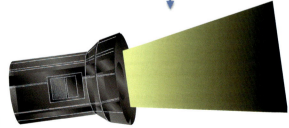

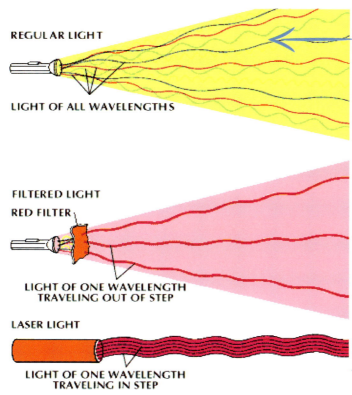

Ordinary wide spectrum white light is composed of different colors and different wavelengths, whereas laser light has one color and collimated wavelength.

Laser's Mechanism of Action

How laser exert its function on tissue?

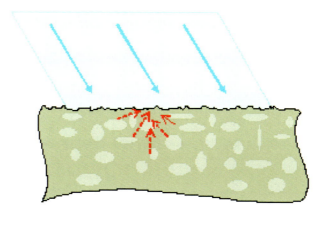

1 - by: Selective Photothermolysis

It is a concept developed by Rox Anderson in 1983.

"Laser light of a specific wavelength can destroy a target containing adequate chromophore without damaging the surrounding tissue."

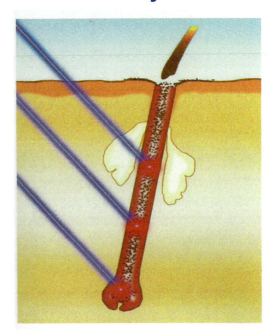

35

1983 Selective Photothermolysis Theory

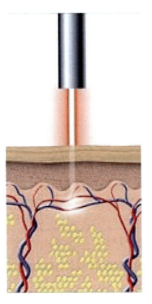

- Energy must penetrate skin and be absorbed by target tissue
- Pulsing of energy must match or be lower than the Thermal Relaxation Time (TRT) of the target
- Must have sufficient energy to have desired effect on target

36

Selective Photothermolysis is possible by the Thermal Relaxation Time.

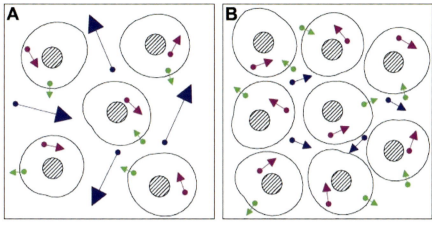

A) Heat outside of cells   B) Diffusion of heat inside the cells

It is the time necessary for a target tissue to cool down by 50% through transfer of heat to surrounding tissue via thermal diffusion.

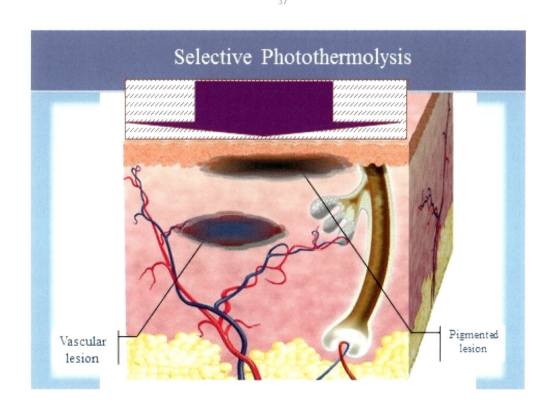

Selective Photothermolysis

Vascular lesion

Pigmented lesion

| Pulsed light heats the melanin in a pigmented lesion, which causes the lesion to disappear. | Specially-filtered pulsed light heats the blood, which damages the lesion and causes it to disappear. |

2 - by: Selective Photocoagulation

Heating process of unwanted blood vessels, skin imperfections and other tissue problems is like a cooking of meat. The heating induced the destabilization of the proteins and enzymes. In this precess the laser radiation heats up tissue above 50°C but below 100°C and induces disordering and denaturing of proteins and other bio-molecules.

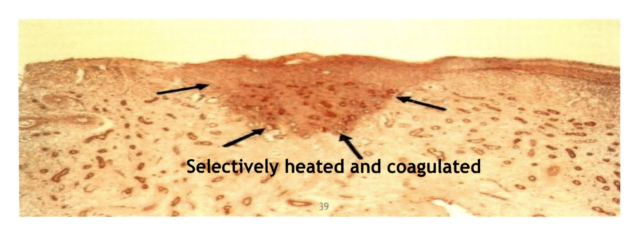

Selectively heated and coagulated

39

Selective Photocoagulation

This process can have effect on and treat, for example, for these conditions:

- Mole Removal
- Capillaries (spider Veins)
- Collagen for skin Tightening

Blood coagulation in a capillary can lead to obstruction and unwanted vein elimination.

40

Laser photocoagulation surgery has been widely used in recent decades to treat a number of eye disorders. During the procedure, a laser beam is utilized to finely cauterize ocular blood vessels.

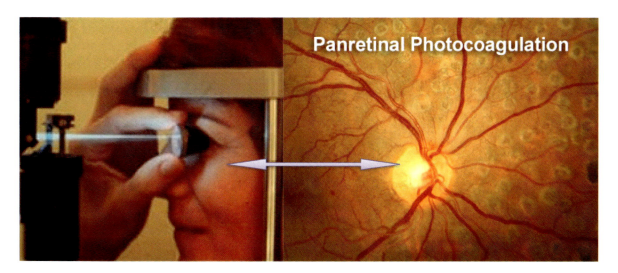

Panretinal Photocoagulation

41

Consequence of photocoagulation

When a laser is used to photocoagulate tissue during surgery, the tissue essentially becomes cooked or denatured:

- The tissue shrinks in mass because water is expelled.
- The heated region change color and loses its mechanical integrity.
- Cells in the photocoagulated region die and a region of dead tissue called photocoagulation burn develops.
- The dead tissue can be removed or pulled out.

42

How laser exerts its function on tissue?

3 - by: Selective Photovaporization

Photo- vaporization results in complete removal of the tissue, making possible for :

Laser Skin Resurfacing

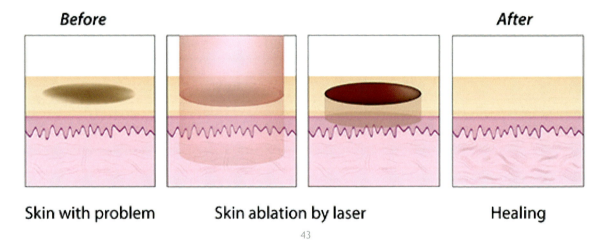

Before   *After*

Skin with problem   Skin ablation by laser   Healing

43

Selective Photovaporization

Using very high power densities, instead of coagulating, the laser will quickly heat the tissue up to above 100 ºC. Then, the water within the tissue instantly boils and evaporates. Since 70% of the body tissue is water, boiling changes the tissue into a gas. This process is known as photovaporization.

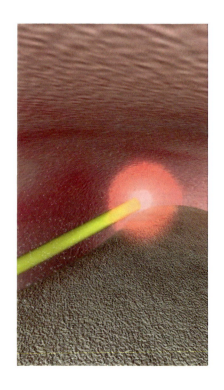

44

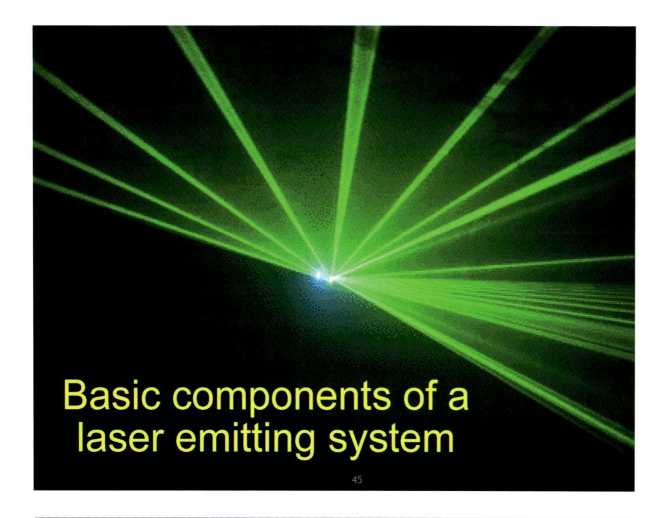

Basic components of a laser emitting system

Basic components of a laser emitting system

There are four basic components to every laser system:

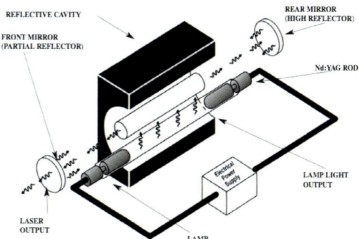

- Optical cavity
- Lasing medium
- Power source
- Delivery system

Basic Elements of a Laser with ND:YAG

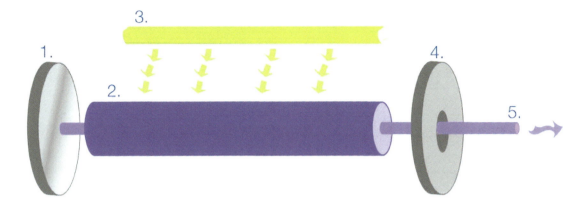

1. Reflective Mirror
2. Nd:YAG crystal rod
3. Flashlamp

4. Output Coupler
5. Laser Beam

Basic components of a laser emitting system: Optical Cavity

Optical Cavity is a chamber located between optics and reflective mirrors that encompasses the lasing medium.

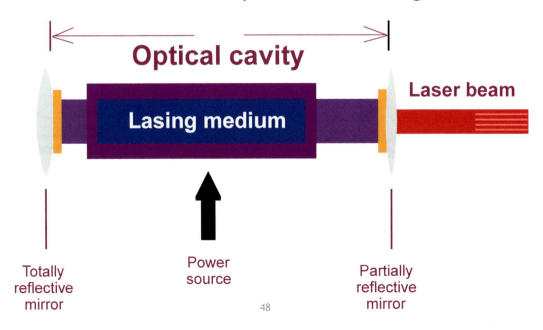

Optical cavity

Lasing medium

Laser beam

Totally reflective mirror

Power source

Partially reflective mirror

SOLID STATE LASER CAVITY

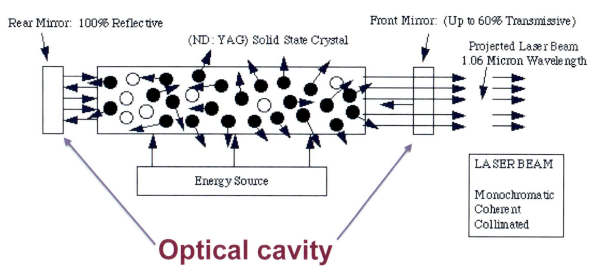

Optical cavity

Optical cavities are major component of lasers, surrounding the gain medium and providing feedback of the laser light. Light confined in the cavity reflects multiple times and produces standing waves for certain resonance frequencies.The optical resonator, or optical cavity, in its simplest form is two parallel mirrors placed around the gain medium which provide feedback of the light. 49

Basic components of a laser emitting system: Lasing Medium

The lasing medium (located inside the optical cavity) is the substance that produces the laser beam. This could be a:

- GAS (Argon, Krypton, CO_2)
- SOLID (Ruby crystals or Alexandrite)
- LIQUID (Dye).

The Lasing Medium determines the wavelength of the laser.

50

Gain medium / Laser medium

The gain medium is the major determining factor of the wavelength of operation and other properties of the laser. Examples of different gain media include:

1 - **Liquids**, such as dye lasers. These are usually organic chemical solvents such as methanol, ethanol or ethylene glycol, to which are added chemical dyes such as coumarin, rhodamine, and fluorescein. The exact chemical configuration of the dye molecules determines the operation wavelength of the dye laser.

2 - **Gases,** such as carbon dioxide, argon, krypton and mixtures such as helium–neon. These lasers are often pumped by electrical discharge.

3 - **Solids,** such as crystals and glasses. The solid host materials are usually doped with an impurity such as chromium, neodymium, erbium or titanium ions. Typical hosts include YAG (yttrium aluminium garnet), YLF (yttrium lithium fluoride), sapphire (aluminium oxide) and various glasses. Examples of solid-state laser media include Nd:YAG, Ti:sapphire, Cr:sapphire (usually known as ruby), Cr:LiSAF (chromium-doped lithium strontium aluminium fluoride), Er:YLF, Nd:glass, and Er:glass. Solid-state lasers are usually pumped by flashlamps or light from another laser.

4 - **Semiconductors,** a type of solid crystal with uniform dopant distribution or material with differing dopant levels in which the movement of electrons can cause laser action. Semiconductor lasers are typically very small, and can be pumped with a simple electric current, enabling them to be used in consumer devices such as compact disc players.

Basic components of a laser emitting system: Power Source

The power source is used to stimulate the Lasing Medium to produce the laser beam.

The power source includes:

- Electricity
- Flash Lamps
- Other Lasers

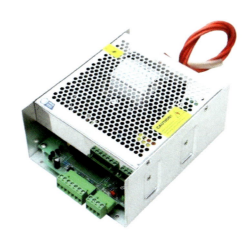

Pump source or Power Source

The pump source is the part that provides energy to the laser system. Examples of pump sources include electrical discharges, flash-lamps, arc lamps, light from another laser, chemical reactions and even explosive devices.

The type of pump source used principally depends on the gain medium, and this also determines how the energy is transmitted to the medium. A helium–neon (HeNe) laser uses an electrical discharge in the helium-neon gas mixture, a Nd:YAG laser uses either light focused from a xenon flash lamp or diode lasers, and excimer lasers use a chemical reaction.

Basic components of a laser emitting System: Delivery System

The delivery system modifies the laser beam and brings it from the optical cavity to the patient.

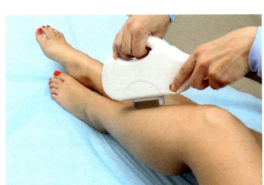

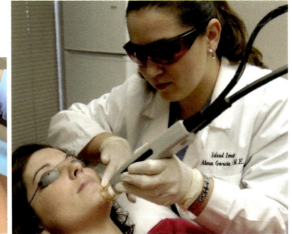

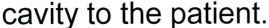
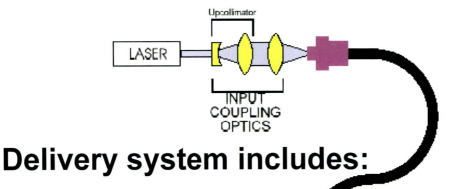
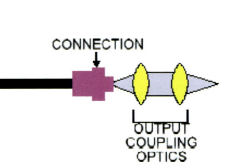

Delivery system includes:

- Articulated arms
- Optical fibers
- Micromanipulators
- Focusing hand-pieces
- Lenses

Light Interaction on Tissue

Light Interaction on Tissue

TYPES OF LASER TREATMENTS

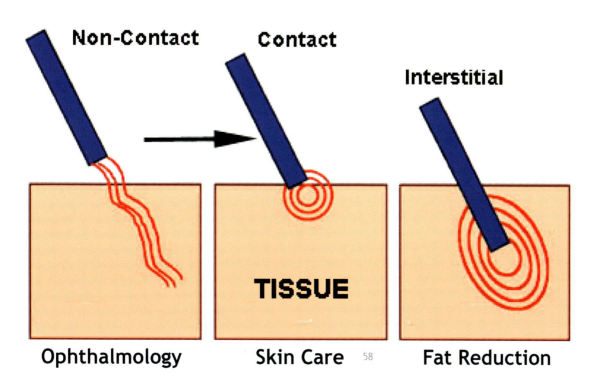

Non-Contact   Contact

Interstitial

TISSUE

Ophthalmology   Skin Care   58   Fat Reduction

Laser vision correction surgery, is a surgical procedure used to correct vision problems that works by reshaping the cornea, or clear front part of the eye, so that light traveling through it is properly focused onto the retina located in the back of the eye.

Non-contact Laser Treatment

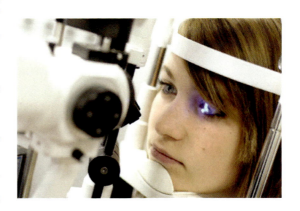

59

Laser resurfacing is a treatment to reduce facial wrinkles and skin irregularities. The technique directs short, concentrated pulsating beams of light at skin, precisely removing skin layer by layer. This popular procedure is also called Lasabrasion, or laser vaporization.

Contact Laser Treatment

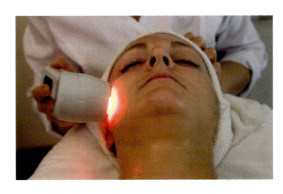

Light Interaction on Tissue

Laser lipolysis, is a non-invasive procedure for the removal of stubborn pockets of fat. It effectively 'melt' the unwanted fat on face and body, then either allows body to metabolize the melted fat or uses aspiration, to remove greater quantities of fat.

Interstitial Laser Treatment

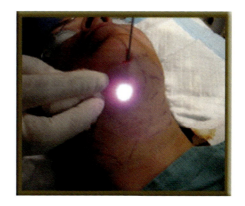

61

Four types of light Interaction on tissue

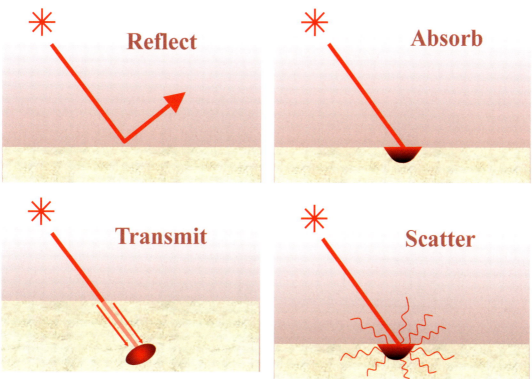

Reflect

Absorb

Transmit

Scatter

62

Desirable Light Interaction on Tissue

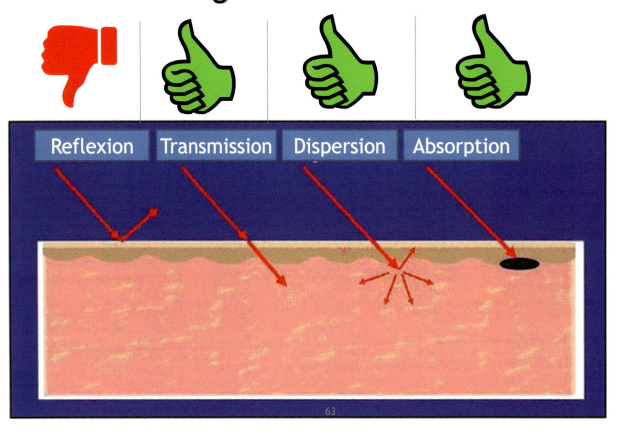

Laser and IPL Adjustment Parameters

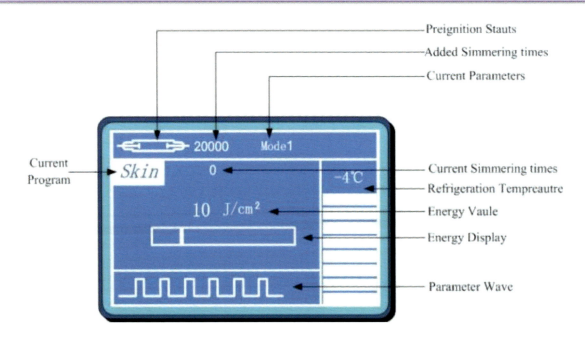

There are four basic laser and IPL parameters:

1. • Wavelength

2. • Pulse duration

3. • Fluence

4. • Spot size

The effect of laser therapy depends on these four parameters.

65

1 - Wavelength

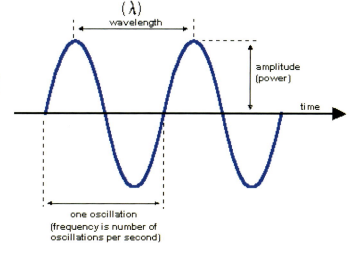

Longer wavelength penetrates deeper into the skin. Conversely, shorter wavelength treats superficial layers of the skin.

66

Wavelength (WL) Strength / Depth of penetration:

Shorter WL   Longer WL

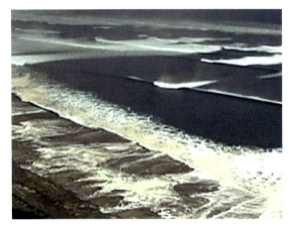
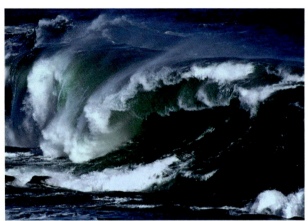

Lower energy   Higher energy

67

Different laser colors have different wavelengths that determine the depth of penetration into the skin.

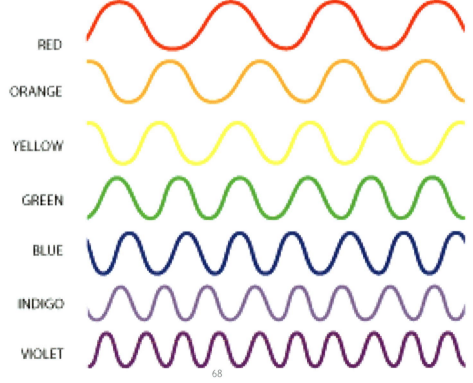

RED

ORANGE

YELLOW

GREEN

BLUE

INDIGO

VIOLET

68

Depth of Penetration by Wavelength

Longer Wavelength penetrates deeper into the skin.

Intense Pulsed Light

Micro-dermabrasion | 2940 Er:YAG | 1440 Nd:YAG | 1540 Er:Glass 1550 Fiber Laser | 585 – 595 Pulse Dye | 694 Ruby | 755 Alexandrite | 810 Diode | 1064 Nd:YAG | 1320 Nd:YAG

69

Laser light depth of penetration

Tissue Penetration

| fd ND: YAG 532 nm | Dye 585 nm | Ruby 694 nm | Alexandrite 755 nm | Diode 800 nm | ND: YAG 1064 nm | Er: YAG 2940 nm | CO$_2$ 10,600 nm |

3 pm   20 pm

Longer wavelength yield to penetration in deeper layers of skin

70

2 - Pulse Duration

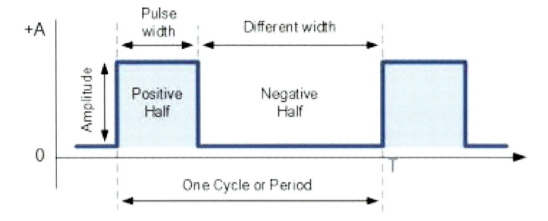

Pulse Duration or Pulse Width is the length of time that a defined amount of energy is delivered to the target tissue.

71

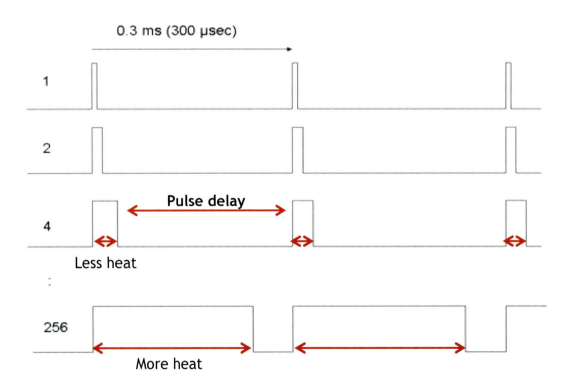

Longer Pulse Duration results in more intense heat.

> Pulse duration (pulse width) refers to the length of each laser pulse.

- **Measured in micro-, milli- or nano-seconds.**

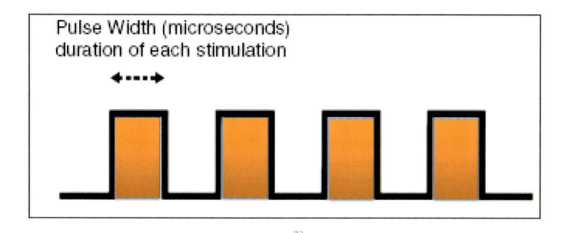

Pulse Width (microseconds)
duration of each stimulation

Laser Pulse Duration

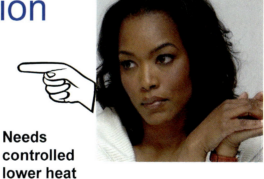

- Shorter pulse duration allows the skin to heat up slower and is safer for darker skin tones.

Needs controlled lower heat

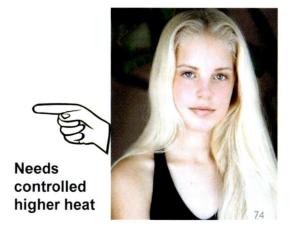

- Longer pulse duration can be more effective for treating fine and light colored hair / white skin.

Needs controlled higher heat

3 - Fluence

Laser Fluence is a measure used to describe the energy delivered per unit or effective area.

(Fluence unit of measurement is J/cm²)

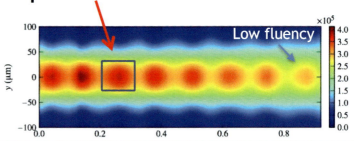

$$\text{Fluence} \left[\frac{\text{Joules}}{\text{cm}^2}\right] = \frac{\text{Laser pulse energy [J]}}{\text{Effective focal spot area [cm}^2\text{]}}$$

75

Fluence

The amount of energy delivered to a given area is referred to "Fluence". Higher Fluence results in higher heat and increased thermal energy. It will achieve better hair removal results, but it may raise the risk of thermal damage and more pain.

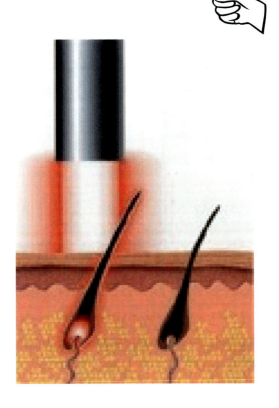

76

The darker the skin	1. Decrease the fluence 2. Increase the pulse delay (allow more cooling)
The lighter the skin	1. Increase the fluence 2. Decrease the pulse delay
The darker the hair / pigmented lesion	1. Decrease the fluence 2. Increase the pulse delay (allow more cooling)
The lighter the hair / pigmented lesion	1. Increase the fluence 2. Decrease the pulse delay
Fine blood vessels	1. higher fluence 2. Decrease the pulse delay 3. Decrease the pulse width
Thicker blood vessels	1. Increase pulse delay (allow more cooling) 2. Increase the pulse width
The smaller the target size / lesion	1. Decrease pulse delay
The larger the target size / lesion	1. Increase pulse delay (allow more cooling)
Bony prominences (forehead, malar area, shins)	1. Decrease the fluence by 10-20%

Laser and IPL Adjustment Parameters

4 - Spot Size

Dimensions of laser / IPL emission size on the hand-peice is referred as spot size.

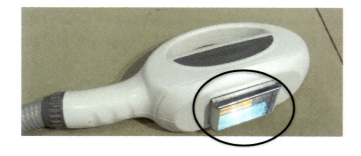 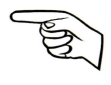

Spot size determines the area to be treated.

Spot Size

A spot size of at least 3-5 mm is suitable for pigmented spots or mole removal but larger spot sizes are required for effective hair removal.

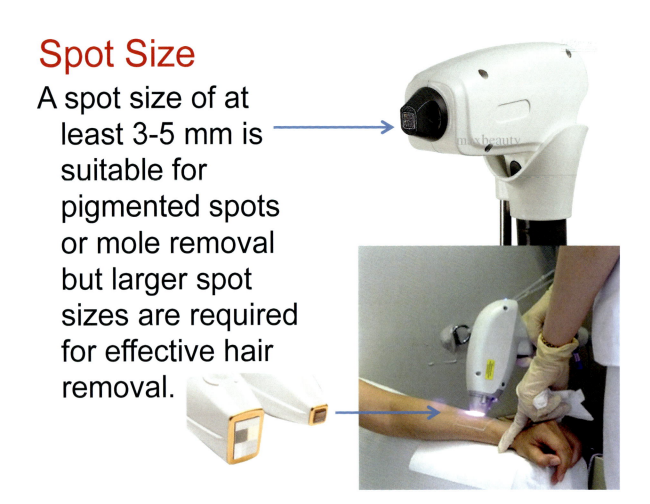

Spot sizes also determine the depth of penetration.

The larger the spot size, the greater the depth of penetration.

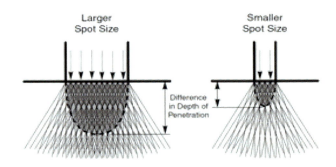

Spot Size Effects in Tissue

- Larger spot size is less affected by scattering than smaller spot size.

- Larger spot size allows for lower fluence level.

- Larger spot size allows deeper penetration in tissue.

81

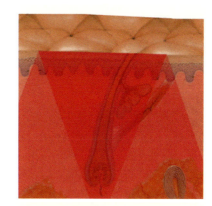

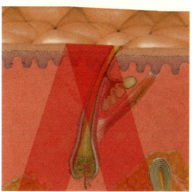

Power Density

Focal distance is important in delivering proper power density to targeted tissue. Holding the hand-piece flat and contacted to skin maintains the power density in a good mode.

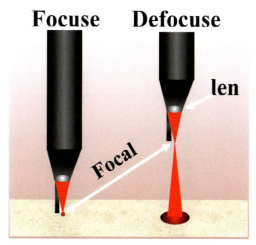

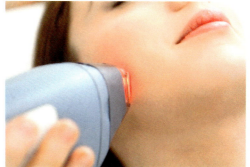

82

TYPES OF COSMETIC AND MEDICAL LASERS

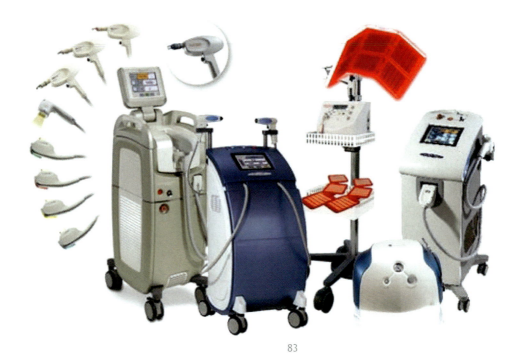

83

Laser machines: types and classifications

Lasers are classified according to a specific range of effectiveness, depending on their:

- Wavelength (penetration)
- Lasing Medium
- Fluence strength
- Application

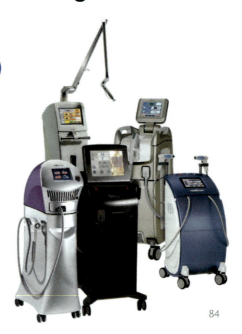

84

TYPES OF COSMETIC / DERMATOLOGY LASERS

There are several different types of medical lasers used in Aesthetic dermatology.

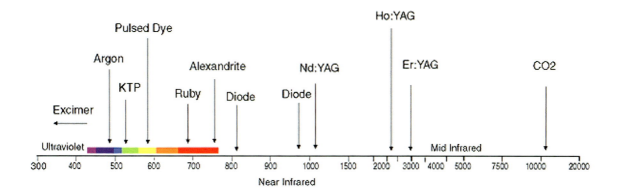

Their effectiveness depends on their wavelength and depth of penetration.

85

Depth of penetration in the skin depends on the wavelength of the laser. Lasers with longer wavelength penetrates deeper.

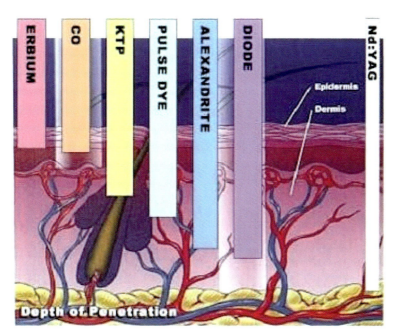

86

What determines the name and type of a Laser Machine?

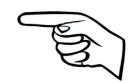

- Lasers are usually named after the amplification materials used.

- For example, the carbon dioxide laser is called a CO2 laser, while the YAG laser contains a solid material made up of Yttrium, Aluminum, and Garnet.

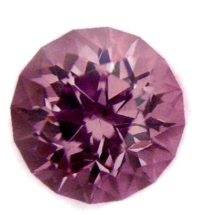

87

Ruby, Alexandrite and Diode lasers, do not penetrate as deep as ND:YAG. They are more effective on superficial targets on skin. YAG laser reaches deeper targets such as hair follicle more efficiently.

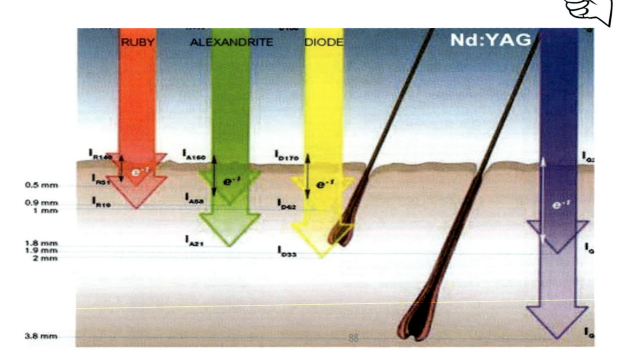

ND:YAG Laser System

Nd:YAG stands for neodymium-doped yttrium aluminium garnet; Nd:$Y_3Al_5O_{12}$, is a crystal that used as a lasing medium for solid-state lasers.

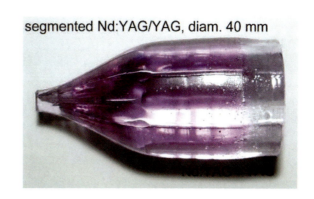
segmented Nd:YAG/YAG, diam. 40 mm

Nd:YAG lasers emitting light at 1064 nm have been widely used for laser-induced thermotherapy, in which benign or malignant lesions in various organs are ablated by the beam.

89

ND:YAG Laser System

ND:YAG is one of the most common types of laser used for many different applications including Cosmetic and Medical purposes.

Nd:YAG lasers can be used to remove skin cancers and other type of malignant tumours.

ND:YAG lasers are also used extensively in the field of cosmetic medicine for laser hair removal and the treatment of minor vascular defects such as spider veins on the face and legs.

90

ND-YAG Laser System

- Provides the maximum output energy of 80 Joules, the highest available in an Nd:YAG laser.

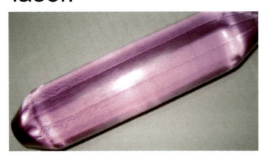

ND:YAG Crystal

- It is absorbed more slowly by both melanin and hemoglobin, ensuring that its energy can penetrate deeply to reach both hair follicles and varicose veins, even in the darkest skin types.

ND:YAG Laser System

ND:YAG has the ability to deliver two different wavelengths of light:

1 - an invisible infrared light used for deeper penetration. This wavelength is used to get to deeper hair follicles.

2 - a green light, is employed for treating hair follicles closer to the surface.

When compared to other lasers, this laser is not that effective on white or light hair and the treatments are quite painful.

ND:YAG Laser System

Suitable for **Skin type V, Skin type VI**

These lasers are used extensively in the field of cosmetic medicine for laser hair removal and the treatment of minor vascular defects such as spider veins on the face and legs.

YAG laser is commonly used to vaporize a portion of the capsule, allowing light to pass through to the retina. The procedure is effective in eliminating the cloudy condition.

93

ND:YAG Laser System

The ND:YAG laser machines can successfully be used on darker skin types with minimal risk.

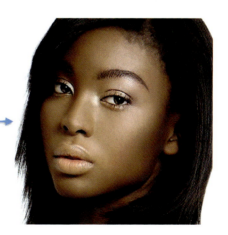

The downside is that, since they are designed to safeguard dark skin from blistering, they are significantly less effectual on fine hairs.

ND:YAG machine is not suitable for white skin.

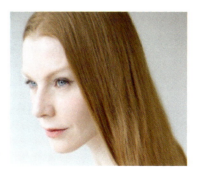

94

RUBY LASER: Wavelength 694 nm

More suitable for **Skin type I, Skin type II**

The Ruby laser is a solid-state laser that uses a synthetic ruby crystal as its gain medium.

This is the oldest type of laser used for hair removal purpose. Ruby laser is suitable for those with fair or white skin and works best for light and fine hair types.

It is not a laser of choice for individuals with tanned or darker skin.

RUBY LASER: Wavelength 694 nm

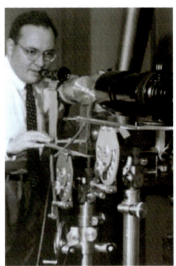

The first working laser was a ruby laser made by Theodore H. "Ted" Maiman at Hughes Research Laboratories on May 16, 1960.

Ruby lasers produce pulses of visible light at a wavelength of 694.3 nm, which is a deep red color.

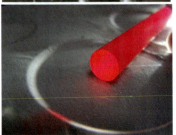

Ruby laser is the original and first system of laser hair removal. It is only suitable for white skins.

The long-term results of Ruby laser hair removal machines are quite well accepted for long term loss of fair hair after treatment.

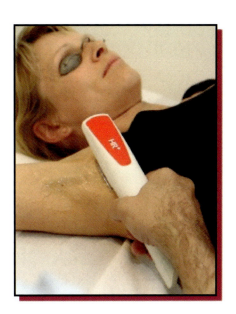

The Ruby laser system is quite old fashioned not as effectual as the newer Alexandrite laser hair removal machines.This laser emits red-colored beam which seeks out the target melanin inside the hair shafts and adjoining hair follicles. The Ruby laser cannot be used on tanned or dark skin and on white or light hair.

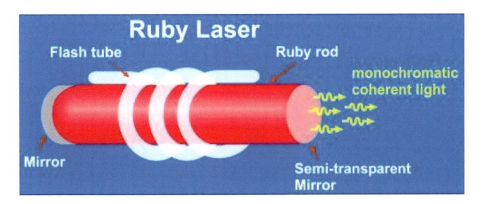

CO2 LASERS: Wavelength 10604 nm

The carbon dioxide laser (CO_2 laser) is one of the most common lasers used in surgery and is good for precise cutting and vaporization of tissue.

CO2 lasers are the highest-power continuous wave lasers that are currently available.

skin resurfacing and dermabrasion that involves thermally inducing the skin to promote collagen formation in the areas of treatment. The CO2 laser is also used by ophthalmic plastic surgeons to remove fine wrinkles from around the eyes.

99

Visible and invisible light and other radiations wavelength on electromagnetic spectrum.

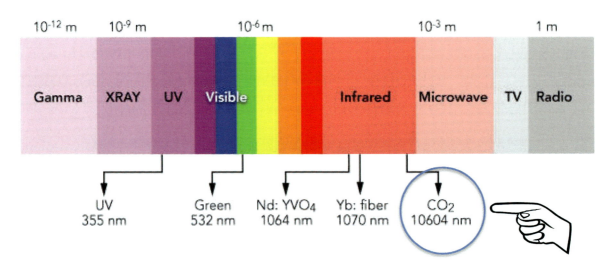

CO2 lasers are the highest-power continuous wave lasers that are currently available.

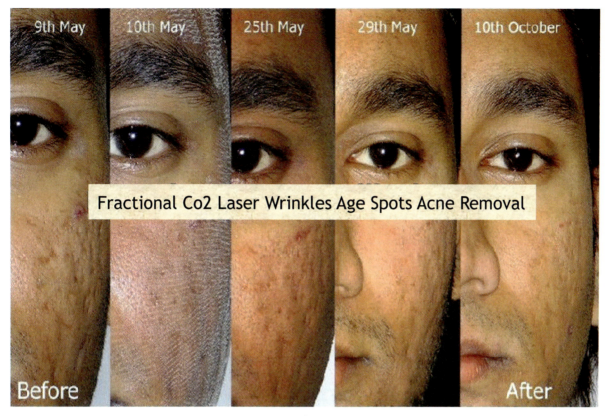

9th May 10th May 25th May 29th May 10th October

Fractional Co2 Laser Wrinkles Age Spots Acne Removal

Before

After

101

ERBIUM LASERS

Erbium lasers produce energy in the mid infrared invisible light spectrum. High degree of absorption enables the laser to precisely and instantly vaporize the target spots in the skin and tissue so that surrounding skin is barely affected. For this reason, Erbium laser has gain popularity due to its painless nature and minimal to no side effects, while the degree of precision and control is significantly enhanced. The Erbium laser is generally used in skin resurfacing and is able to remove finer wrinkles with less damage to the skin.

ERBIUM LASERS: wavelength of 2940 nm

Erbium lasers produce energy in the mid infrared invisible light spectrum that is better absorbed up to 15 times by water in the skin than the energy from CO2 lasers.

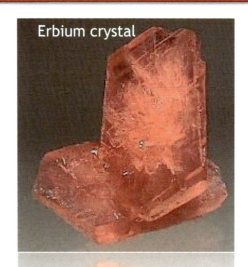

Erbium crystal

This fact limits the use of this laser in surgery, and in many other laser applications where the water is present. Erbium lasers emit infrared light with a wavelength of 2940 nm.

ERBIUM LASERS: wavelength of 2940 nm

Erbium laser has gain popularity due to its painless nature and minimal to no side effects for skin laser resurfacing.

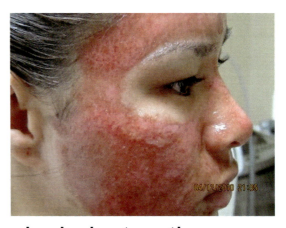

Example of applications include treating acne scarring, deep rhytides, and melasma. The output of ER lasers is also absorbed by hydroxyapatite, which makes it a good laser for cutting bone as well as soft tissue.

ERBIUM vs. CO2 LASERS

Erbium laser is considered to be more precise and accurate than the CO2 laser. The depth of Erbium laser penetration is about 5 microns compared with the 20 microns typical of the CO2 laser. The Erbium laser has also been shown to cause less uneven skin pigmentation in darker skinned individuals since it creates a thinner laser area and less heat. Erbium laser also has minimal heat diffusion and reduced tissue thermal damage, therefore, it has lower healing time than that within the CO2 laser. The Erbium laser is also being used in a promising new clinical procedure to emulsify the eye's natural lens during cataract surgery. Most cataract surgeons currently use a piece of equipment called a phacoemulsifier to break up and remove the cloudy lens. The Erbium laser was chosen for the new technique because of its high absorption rate in water, a primary component of the eye's natural crystalline lens. 105

ALEXANDRITE Laser: Wavelength 755 nm

Most suitable for Skin type I, type II, type III

Alexandrite laser is most appropriate for the treatment of dermal pigmented lesions. This laser is known to be effective on finer, thinner hairs that other lasers are not effective with.

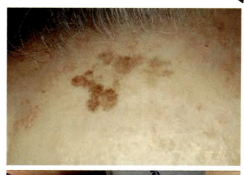

The Alexandrite laser hair removal systems are traditionally highly effectual for white-skinned, dark-haired patients. 106

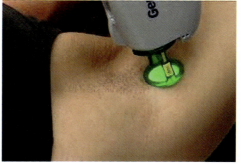

ALEXANDRITE Laser: Wavelength 755 nm

The long-pulse Alexandrite laser has the ability of penetrate deep into the dermis which enables it to achieve effective laser hair removal.

The disadvantages with this laser is that it may cause pigment changes (darkening or lightening) of the skin and is not suitable for darker skin tones.

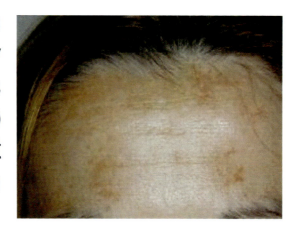

107

ALEXANDRITE & Q-SWITCHED LASERS

Quality-switched systems in which ultra-short bursts (10 to 100 ns) of stored high energy are produced include the 694-nm ruby laser, the 755-nm alexandrite laser and the 1064 – nm Nd:YAG laser. The longer wavelength of these lasers makes them most appropriate for the treatment of dermal pigmented lesions. Q-switching, which is often called giant pulse formation, occurs when a laser creates high-powered pulses of light. The result is a laser beam that emits pulses of light that extremely concentrated and powerful.

DIODE LASERS: Wavelength 800 nm

Suitable for all Skin types: I, II, III, IV.

The diode laser is a proficient machine made up of tiny diodes or semiconductors assembled together to produce light.

The diode laser has a longer wavelength than the Alexandrite and Ruby lasers and thus is able to penetrate deeper into the skin, allowing treatment on dark-skinned people as well as on white-skinned patients.

109

DIODE LASERS: Wavelength 800 nm

In a diode laser the active medium is a semiconductor similar to that found in a light-emitting diode. The way Diode Laser Hair Removal works is based on selective photo thermolysis. When the laser beams are projected on to the specific chromophore area, the energy of the beams heats up the pigment melanin in the hair follicle. Devices, which are most commonly employed in this method, include the SLP 100, F1 Diode, Light Sheer, MeDioStar, LaserLite, Epistar and Apex 800. Because this laser uses a longer wavelength of light in its working, it is more effective on people with darker skin.

110

PULSED DYE LASERS

A dye laser uses an organic dye as the lasing medium, usually as a liquid solution. Compared to gases and most solid state lasting media, a dye can usually be used for a much wider range of Wavelength. The wide range of frequencies makes them particularly suitable for pulsed lasers. In addition, the dye can be replaced by another type in order to generate different wavelengths with the same laser, although this usually requires replacing other optical components in the laser as well.

PULSED DYE LASERS

Dye lasers are very versatile. In addition to their recognized wavelength agility, these lasers can offer very large pulsed energies or very high average powers. Flash-lamp-pumped dye lasers have been shown to yield hundreds of Joules per pulse and copper-laser-pumped dye lasers are known to yield average powers in the kilowatt regime. The pulsed dye laser delivers energy at a wavelength and duration that has been optimized for the selective treatment of vascular lesions. Pulsed dye lasers have been used as an alternative to surgical excision or carbon dioxide lasers.

Intense pulsed light is based on the use of incoherent light over a range of wavelengths from 400 nm to 1200 nm. Xenon flashlamps produce high output bursts of broad spectrum.

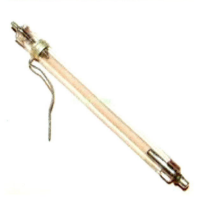

A flashlamp, is an electric lamp designed to produce extremely intense, full-spectrum white light for very short durations. It is made of a length of glass tubing with electrodes at either end and are filled with a gas that, when triggered, ionizes and conducts a high voltage pulse to produce the light.

113

IPL stands for Intense Pulsed Light

Suitable for all Skin types: I, II, III, IV, V and a variety of treatments.

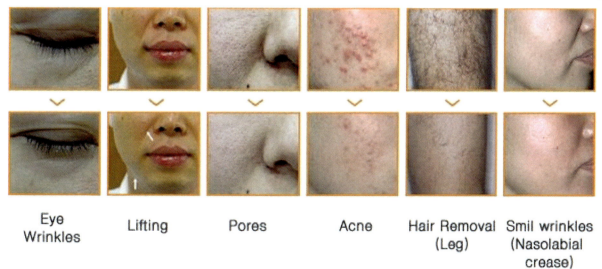

| Eye Wrinkles | Lifting | Pores | Acne | Hair Removal (Leg) | Smil wrinkles (Nasolabial crease) |

IPL: Wavelength 400 - 1200 nm

IPL white light comprises a wide range of colors and wavelengths.

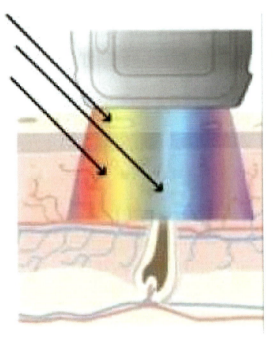

The polychromatic light can reach multiple chromophores in human skin: mainly hemoglobin, water, and melanin. This results in selective photothermolysis of the target, which can be blood vessels, pigmented cells, or hair follicles.

IPL: Wavelength 400 - 1200 nm

Laser only has one color and specific wavelength and depth of penetration into the skin layers.

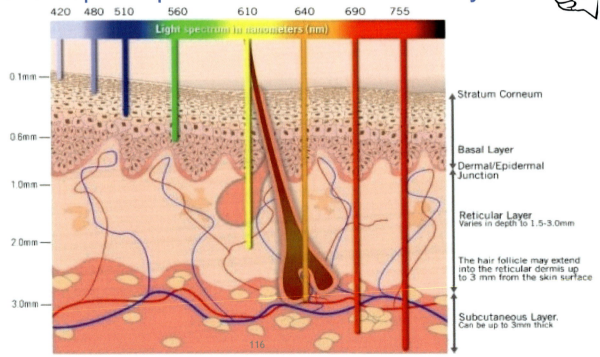

Differences between Laser and IPL

IPL uses a wide spectrum of wavelengths at the same time (for example: 400nm — 1200nm) that can target any chromophore in that range.

Lasers have one wavelength (for example: 800nm) with a very specific target.

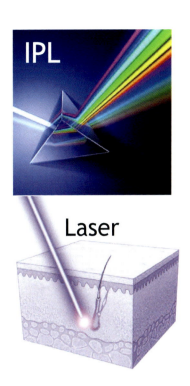

Laser can precisely hit a single target with one shot, whereas, IPL can hit several targets at once.

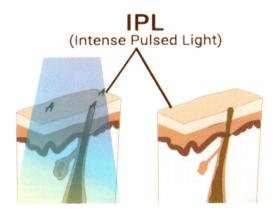

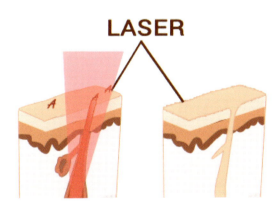

Different wavelengths penetrate the skin to different depths so using IPL is like using a group of lasers in a single treatment.

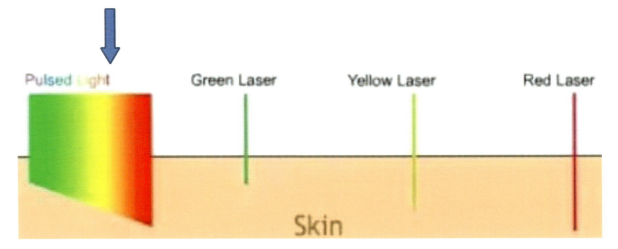

Using IPL, the area that can be treated is larger and the treatment is faster.

IPL uses special filters that block unwanted wavelengths. The filters can be changed to "cut off" the shorter wavelengths. The appropriate filter will depend on the depth of the intended target.

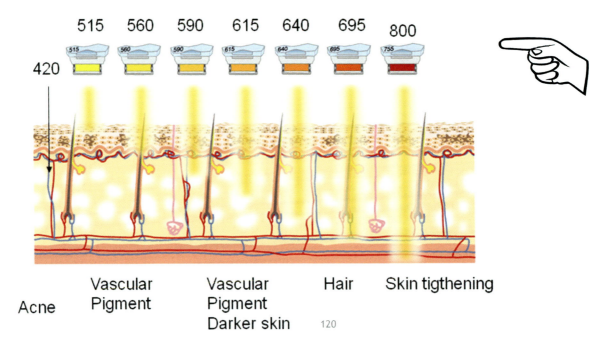

IPL is well absorbed by chromophores that have color such as melanin, hemoglobin. The concentration of a specific chromophore peaks at different depths in the skin.

The filter used in treatment is decided based on the depth of a desired target and the color of skin. A deeper cut off filter would be used for hair removal, while a shallow filter would be used when treating vascular issues such as rosacea.

Patients with darker skin should seek treatment from experienced practitioners in treating their skin type, to avoid complications. 121

Laser / IPL Machine Cooling System

The temperature exposed to melanin pigment may be increased in the hair follicle beyond its capacity and / or dispersed into the surrounding structures. Cooling mechanisms are needed to prevent thermal damage or burns.

Laser light is converted to thermal energy when reaches the target through diffusion of heat during skin laser therapy.

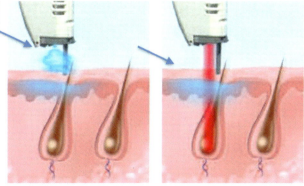

Since laser's light is converted to thermal energy when reach the target, cooling mechanisms are needed to prevent thermal damage or burns. Therefore, most lasers device in medical aesthetics are equipped with a cooling mechanism necessary enough to prevent damage to the surrounding cells where no treatment is needed. Generally, through diffusion of heat during skin laser therapy the temperature exposed to melanin pigment may be increased in the hair follicle beyond its capacity and / or dispersed into the surrounding structures. Cooling mechanisms protect the surface of the skin and decrease the risk of blistering and unwanted pigment alteration. In addition, it causes less pain, swelling and more effective results. Generation of extreme heat in darkly pigmented skin can also be controlled effectively with cooling mechanisms.

Laser / IPL Machine Cooling System

There are several basic types of cooling mechanisms used with lasers.

- Cryogen- cooling systems
- Air- cooling systems
- Water Contact cooling systems

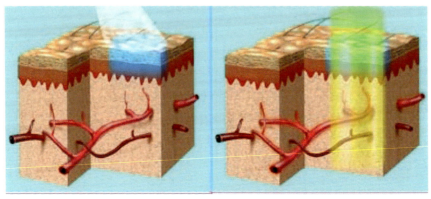

Laser / IPL Machine Cooling System

There are several basic types of cooling mechanisms used with lasers. Cryogen-, Air- and Contact-cooling systems are examples of advanced technology with minimal adverse effects. Cryogen spray is a most common method of cooling in lasers. Cryogen is a refrigerant at -30 to -50°C that is sprayed onto the skin before and/or after laser irradiation. It distributes consistent and effective cooling on the skin treated laser however, in addition to being costly, excess cryogen spray may cause skin freezing and blisters. Water-cooling mechanism can be an effective alternative with minimal side effects.

Laser / IPL Machine Cooling System

Application of cooling gels is the least effective cooling mechanisms due to uneven distribution of the gel during procedure and potentially insufficient cooling. It also provides short-term, superficial effectiveness and may be unpleasant to some users. Contact-cooling can be very accurate and effective. This method uses a cold gliding hand piece over a gel. The most important consideration for a client in a medical aesthetics setting is to choose an experienced cosmetic physician or licensed technician who is knowledgeable in the different laser and cooling methods. The laser operators must also be very skillful with the technique used, especially if contact cooling is the preferred cooling method.

Cryogen spray is a most common method of cooling in lasers. Cryogen is a refrigerant at -30 to -50°C that is sprayed onto the skin before and/or after laser irradiation.

Cryogen sprayed onto skin milliseconds before laser pulse. Epidermis is optimally protected during laser pulse

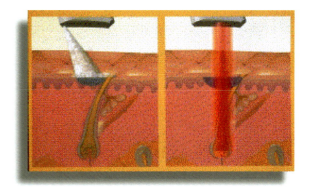

127

Air-cooling system can be an effective alternative with minimal side effects.

Cold air is blown to the treatment area from the laser wand to reduce the risk of thermal damage.

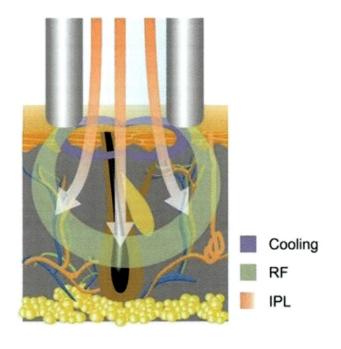

Cooling

RF

IPL

128

- Application of cooling gels is the least effective cooling mechanisms due to uneven distribution of the gel during procedure and potentially insufficient cooling.

- Contact-cooling can be very accurate and effective. This method uses a cold gliding hand piece over a gel.

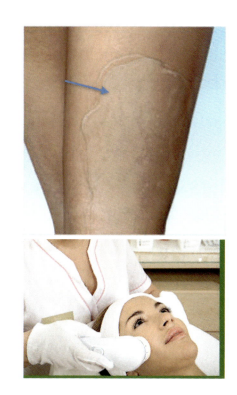

129

Safety for Cosmetic Laser Procedures for skin care

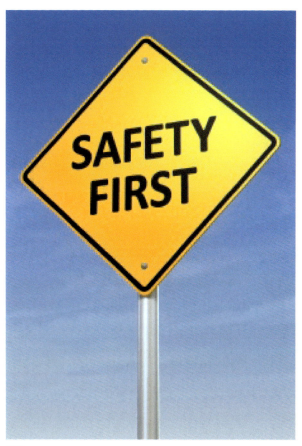

130

Laser operation safety measures in a skin care clinic

Even short, accidental exposure to high-power laser radiation can cause permanent eye injury and/or skin burns. When a person chooses to work in a clinic that offer cosmetic or medical laser treatment, it is important for that person to be aware of the hazards involved and the safeguards to protect their clients, themselves and others. This chapter is designed to give owners and operating staff of laser devices essential information for laser safety.

Laser operation safety measures in a skin care clinic

However, simply following the guidelines listed in this book does not relieve the owner or operator from the obligation to take any additional measures necessary to prevent health hazards from occurring in the establishment. Operators should refer to the user information supplied by the manufacturer or distributor of their equipment, as well as any training resource materials and related guidance documents. Owners are also responsible for ensuring that they carry on business in compliance with municipal and provincial regulatory requirements, and for obtaining business licences and/or operating permits from the appropriate licensing authorities.

Most Common Laser Accidents

1. Exposure during alignment -most frequent cause
2. Misaligned optics and stray beams
3. Improper methods of handling high voltage
4. Use of incorrect eyewear or eyewear failure
5. Improper restoration of equipment after service
6. Inhalation of laser generated materials

Laser operation safety measures in a skin care clinic

Lasers used for skin rejuvenation and hair removal are safe to use when specific guidelines are followed. Laser systems are extremely powerful and all precautions must be taken to prevent unintentional exposure to the skin or eyes of direct or indirect reflected laser beam. The wavelength for lasers used in cosmetic skin procedures can pass through glass or windows and can be reflected off metallic surfaces. Even though some of the lasers may use invisible light, it can cause permanent damage. Both the operator and the patient must wear protective eyewear appropriate for the wavelength emitted by the machine.

Laser operation safety measures in a skin care clinic

Even with protective eyewear, it is advisable never to look directly into the hand piece, laser beam, or scattered light from reflective surfaces. It is now standard of care to avoid laser treatments around the eye, including eyebrows.Treatment room doors should remain closed during the operation to prevent accidental exposure. Treatment room windows and portholes should be covered with material of sufficient optical density to prevent laser light from escaping. Reflective objects, such as mirrors, should be removed from the treatment room.

Laser operation safety measures in a skin care clinic

Warning signs should be posted in prominent locations. The exterior housing of a laser should never be removed, except by an authorized service representative. Extremely high voltages can cause fatal shock. It is possible for the high voltage components to retain charge even after the laser has been turned off. Oxygen and flammable substances should not be stored in laser room. This includes alcohol, acetone and flammable anesthetics. Patients must always remember to wear the appropriate eyewear provided to them and never take it off unless advised.

IPL / Laser requires eye protection

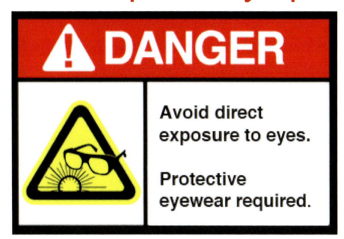

⚠ DANGER

Avoid direct exposure to eyes.

Protective eyewear required.

Eyewear is the single most important piece of protective equipment needed by persons within the laser treatment controlled area. Studies have shown that 70 % of laser eye accidents resulted simply because available protective eyewear was not worn, or inappropriate/ damaged eyewear was worn.

137

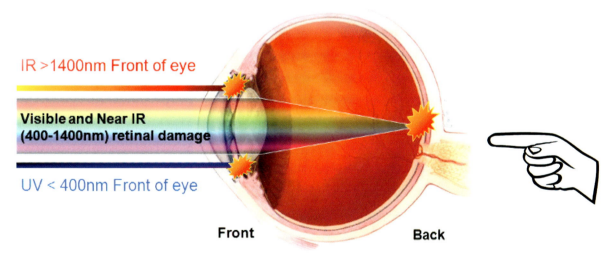

IR >1400nm Front of eye

Visible and Near IR (400-1400nm) retinal damage

UV < 400nm Front of eye

Front   Back

The most important factor in selecting operator protective eyewear is that it must protect against the wavelength emitted by the laser. Protective eyewear must be labelled with the same wavelength that is emitted by the laser (i.e. 755 nm, 810 nm, 1064 nm, etc).

138

Depending on the wavelength of the laser system in operation, an accidental radiation to the eyes can result in potential damage to specific eye anatomy.

- UV - chemical, damage to 1st 20 microns of eye surface.

- Visible and IR Near – damage to internal components of eye (retina). i.e: Nd:YAG, Holmium YAG, Erbium YAG, Erbium Glass.

-

- IR Far - ablative, damage to surface of eye or cornea (CO_2 Laser).

Laser Safety Eyewear

should be labeled with O.D. and wavelength. Protective eyewear for both operator and the patient should to be able to stop laser radiation coming from all directions to prevent striking the eyes. Laser protective eyewear for the laser operator must also allow visible light to pass through so that the wearer can see adequately to perform the tasks safely, while at the same time preventing the wavelength emitted by the laser from passing through.

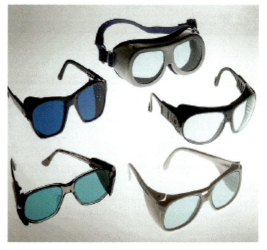

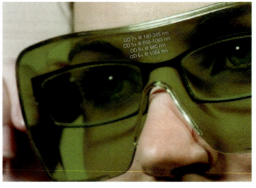

Control of Laser Hazards:

- Accidental Reflection must be prevented by covering or removing of:

- Mirrors

- Jewelries

- Window glasses

  All unnecessary reflective items and shiny tools, extra mirrors, jewelry, watch, plastic ID card, etc.) must be removed from the work table.

Indirect Laser is harmful to eyes even if it is reflected

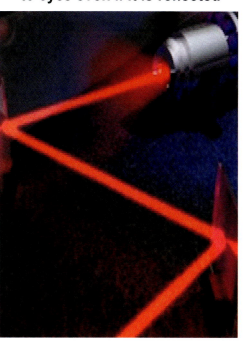

141

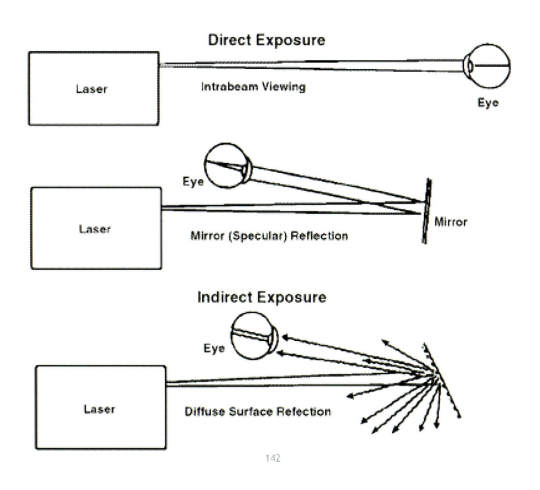

142

Classification of Laser Beam Hazards

- <u>Class I</u>: No known biological hazard
- <u>Class II</u>: Chronic viewing hazard only
- <u>Class III</u>: Direct viewing hazard
- <u>Class IV</u>: Direct and reflected hazard

Two types of eye injury by laser radiation

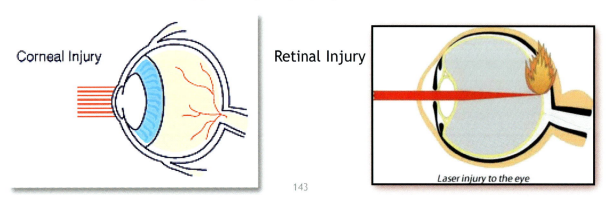

143

ANSI standards for eye safety:

Class III: Helium-neon

- Dangerous only if viewed directly

Class IV: Dye, Nd: YAG, Alexandrite, Diode

- Dangerous to view

- Scattered radiation

- Goggles mandatory

1) Helium-neon lasers are class III. Dye, Nd:YAG, Alexandrite, Diode are class IV lasers and are dangerous to view due to scattered radiation. Use of goggles is mandatory.

2) All windows in a laser treatment room should be protected from beam transmission and covered with opaque material. There should be no mirrors in the treatment room.

3) All doors to a laser treatment room are to be closed and have a laser specific danger sign along with a pair of laser eyewear prominently displayed.

4) Eyes of patients and healthcare workers should be protected from laser beams. Laser-safe eye protection with appropriate wavelength and optical density should be worn by all health care workers and all patients and labeled to protect against improper use.

5) CO_2 Erbium Diode exposure may result in corneal absorption, while Pulsed dye, Nd:YAG, and Alexandrite exposure may result in retinal absorption.

6) Patient eyewear choices include opaque tanning bed eyewear, laser eyewear with proper wavelength protection and optical density, or in the event neither are available; alternatives eye protection may include moist sponges or a wet towel.

7) Flammable or combustible materials such as anesthetics solutions, drying agents, ointments, plastics, and resins, should not be exposed to laser beam.

8) A laser should always be in standby mode unless an operator is ready to use it.

9) How to deal with Plume: A plume is any smoke by-product from the lasers thermal destruction of tissue (may include skin, blood, or viral particles) and may be hazardous to one's respiratory tract. Plume can contain toxic gases and vapours such as benzene, hydrogen cyanide and formaldehyde, bio-aerosols, dead and live cellular materials including blood fragments and viruses. A laser protective mask (0.1 micron) should be used to decrease inhalation of particulate matter. 147

Laser Treatment Controlled Areas, Warning Signs, & Engineering Controls

To ensure that individuals are not exposed to direct, reflected or scattered laser radiation without appropriate protection, it is necessary to:

- Create a "laser treatment controlled area within the facility.

- Install adequate engineering controls.

- Post appropriate warning signs.

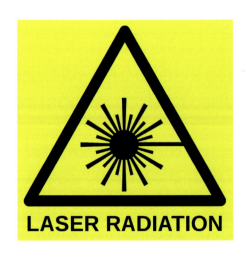

LASER RADIATION

148

All rooms in which lasers are operated must be posted with permanent door-type laser warning signs that include all information appropriate to the lasers operated within the rooms (e.g., laser types and classes, output characteristics).

Doorknob-type warning signs ("Do not enter", "Laser operating inside") should be temporarily posted.

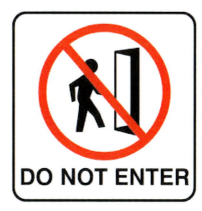

149

Laser Treatment Controlled Areas, Warning Signs, & Engineering Controls

Sign dimensions, letter size and color, etc. must be in accordance with American National Standard Specification for Accident Prevention Signs, ANSI Z535 series. For Class 3B or 4 lasers, the following is required: The signal word "DANGER"

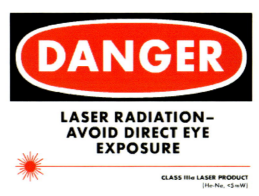

150

Fire hazards

Class 4 visible and infrared beams with irradiance above 10 W/cm2 can ignite combustible beam enclosure materials. Keep combustible materials, including organic solvents, away from laser use areas. Never use cardboard or paper for high power visible or infrared beam containment.

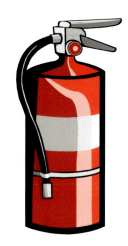

151

Control of Laser Hazards: Non - Beam Hazards

- Fire Safety
- Electrical Safety
- Certified & trained operators
- Sanitizing Station & Solutions
- No unauthorized access
- Laser signes
- Laser room ventilation
- No unnecessary idling
- Stand by mode in effect

152

Chemical hazards

Fluorine and chlorine gases are used with excimer lasers. These need to be stored in approved ventilated gas cabinets. Dye solutions used with dye lasers need to be mixed in a properly functioning fume hood by personnel wearing a lab coat, impermeable gloves, and chemical safety eyewear. Material Safety Data sheets for toxic materials must be reviewed prior to usage.

Laser-generated air contaminants

These are potentially-toxic substances generated when high power laser beams strike target materials (plastic, tissue, etc.). General / dilution ventilation and local exhaust ventilation are two means of controlling this hazard. In some cases respirators need to be worn.

153

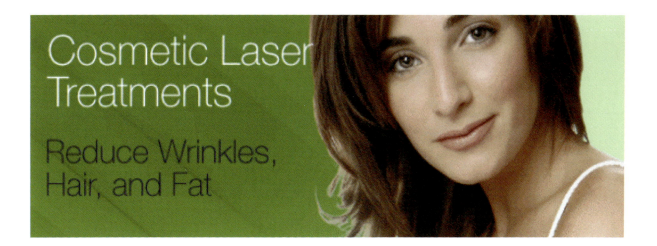

Cosmetic Laser Treatments

Reduce Wrinkles, Hair, and Fat

Procedures that you can perform with a Laser / IPL System

154

Procedures that you can perform with a Laser / IPL System

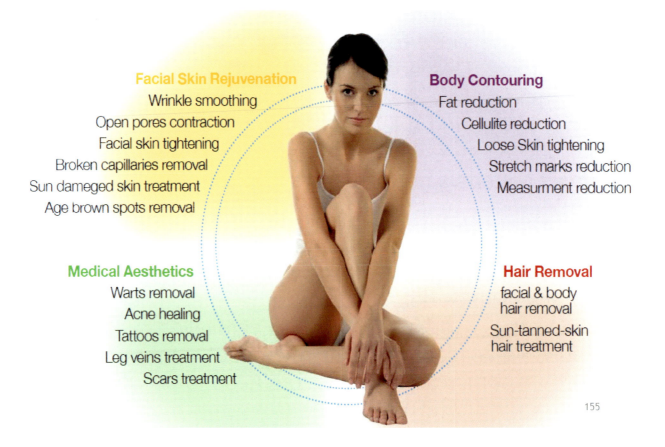

Facial Skin Rejuvenation
Wrinkle smoothing
Open pores contraction
Facial skin tightening
Broken capillaries removal
Sun dameged skin treatment
Age brown spots removal

Body Contouring
Fat reduction
Cellulite reduction
Loose Skin tightening
Stretch marks reduction
Measurment reduction

Medical Aesthetics
Warts removal
Acne healing
Tattoos removal
Leg veins treatment
Scars treatment

Hair Removal
facial & body
hair removal
Sun-tanned-skin
hair treatment

155

1 - Skin Tightening:

Most cosmetic lasers provide some level of superficial tightening at the least, because they produce a controlled injury of the skin, which shrinks the loose collagen and encourages increased collagen production.

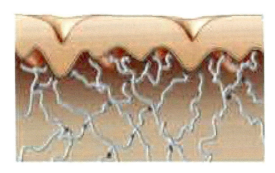

BEFORE

156

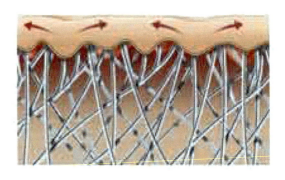

AFTER

Skin tightening by inducing controlled wounding in the dermis results in tissue shrinkage within 2 days and new collagen formation in 4 weeks.

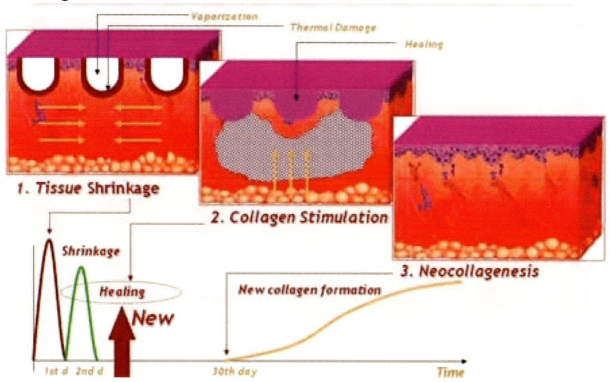

Skin tightening around neck by Intense Pulsed Light / Laser treatment

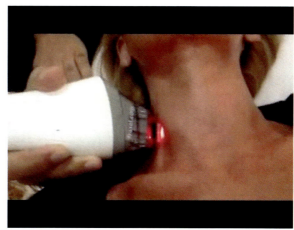

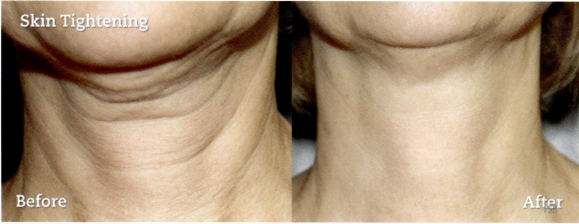

Skin Tightening by new collagen formation:

It is shown that laser treatment stimulate fibroblasts, skin cells that are responsible for collagen production, to synthesize new collagen at the areas of treatment.

Pre Treatment

Post Treatment

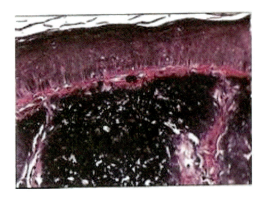
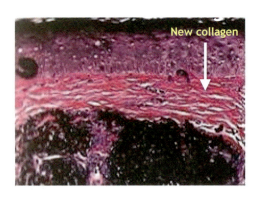

Photos show the collagen growth smoothening and firming the skin.

159

Skin Tightening under the eyes:

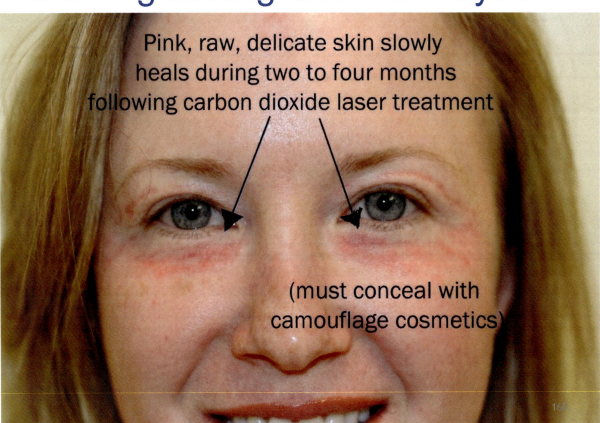

Pink, raw, delicate skin slowly heals during two to four months following carbon dioxide laser treatment

(must conceal with camouflage cosmetics)

Skin Tightening and facial wrinkle reduction by Fractional Laser Therapy

Before   After six session

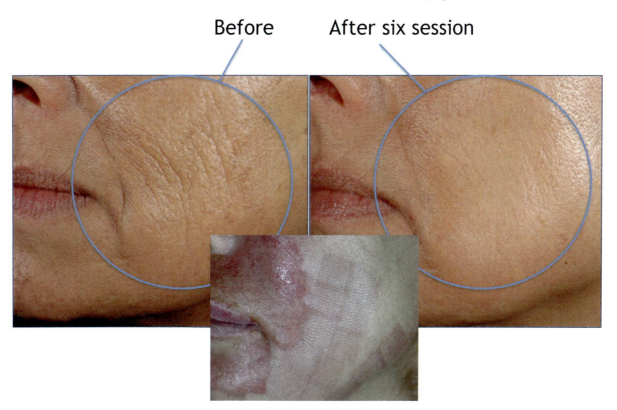

Skin Tightening by IPL / Laser

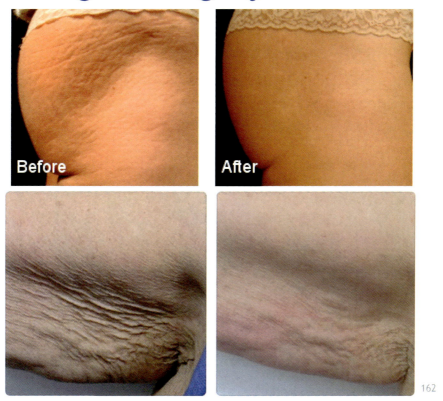

Before   After

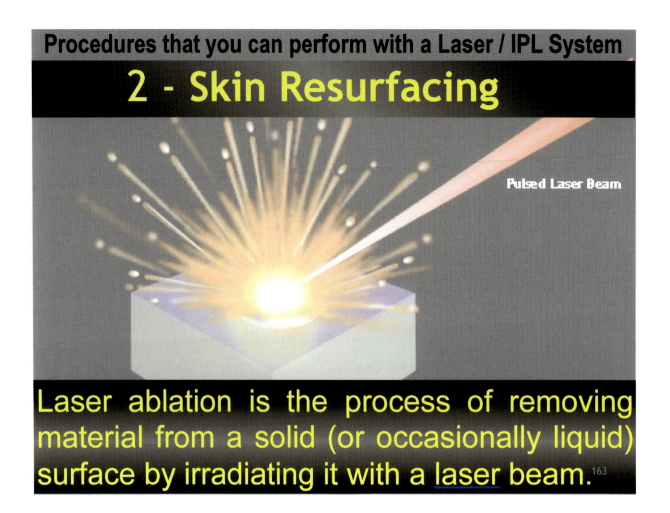

2 - Skin Resurfacing

Pulsed Laser Beam

Laser ablation is the process of removing material from a solid (or occasionally liquid) surface by irradiating it with a laser beam.[163]

LASER SKIN RESURFACING

Laser resurfacing is a major rejuvenation procedure. It is an efficient and inexpensive way to refurbish the younger appearance and freshness to the aged skin. The most preferred benefits of laser skin resurfacing are the considerable diminution of wrinkles, obliterating skin blemishes, and eliminating the sun damage, and age and sun spots. Certain types of scarring and most medium depth wrinkles can be dramatically reduced with laser rejuvenation. Laser eyelid surgery also has become more popular since treats tired, baggy eyes, drooping eyelids, wrinkles, crow's feet, puffiness and dark circles with less bleeding and swelling and less risk of scarring compared to traditional surgical procedure.

LASER SKIN RESURFACING

Skin resurfacing works by removing the outmost layers of skin, epithelium until the wrinkles or scars are eliminated. Most clients can feel a fresh and rejuvenated skin in 3 to 5 days after the treatment when re-epithelialization process is completed and new epithelium grows again. The procedure requires skill and the ability to follow up with the patient in order to avoid any complications.Two types of lasers used for skin rejuvenation are called ablative and non-ablative. The ablative lasers are those, which utilize carbon dioxide - erbium also known, as micro laser peels are very powerful lasers that remove the outermost layer of the skin up to 0.1 mm or 100 microns. Erbium:YAG Laser in combination with the CO2 Laser delivers a short burst of extremely high energy laser light. 165

LASER SKIN RESURFACING

The treatment requires one to two weeks healing process after which skin rejuvenation is satisfactorily achieved by a smoother tighter appearance. After healing, there is a pink to red color that will fade over a few weeks to months. One of the advantages of Erbium laser is preciseness that allows the depth of penetration is highly controlled. The Erbium is highly absorbed by tissue water and less heat is transmitted to the surrounding tissue. People with wide range of skin characteristics including darker skin can be treated with this type of laser. This procedure requires determination of the skin type and highly experienced practitioner to set the device appropriately for skin resurfacing.

Ablative vs. non-ablative laser skin resurfacing

Non-ablative procedures are minimal to no downtime procedures, while ablative procedures provide a single treatment option.

Unlike ablative lasers, which remove the top layer of skin and part of the sub-layer, non-ablative fractional lasers keep the outer layer of skin in place, for faster healing and recovery.

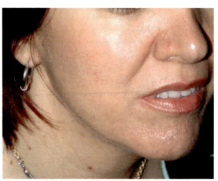

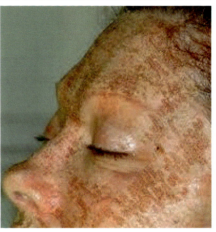

167

Ablative vs non-ablative laser therapy for skin resurfacing and rejuvenation

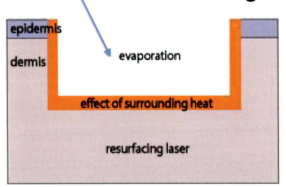

epidermis

dermis

evaporation

effect of surrounding heat

resurfacing laser

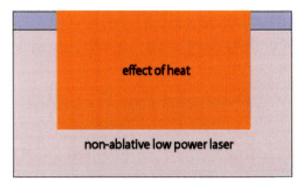

effect of heat

non-ablative low power laser

In nonablative laser treatments the skin surface remains largely intact.

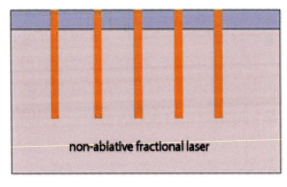

non-ablative fractional laser

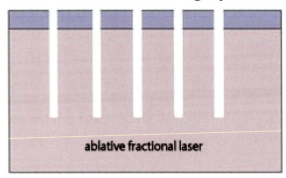

ablative fractional laser

Ablative laser skin resurfacing:

A process where the upper layers of aged or damaged skin are vaporized by heat from applying a controlled laser therapy.

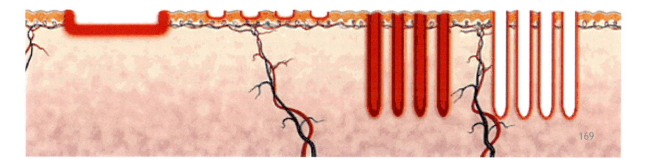

Ablative Resurfacing	Superficial Fractional Ablative Resurfacing	Non-Ablative Fractional Resurfacing	Ablative Fractional Resurfacing
10-200 mircons	10-70 mircrons	600-1000 microns	600-1000 microns

Skin Regeneration Process
After Fractional CO2 Laser

Immediately After Laser	**Post 2 days**	**Post 14 days**
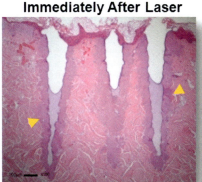	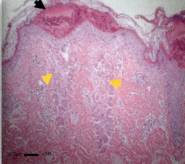	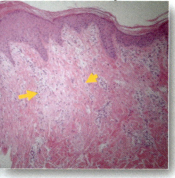
▪Ablated epidermis and dermis	▪Re-epithelialization and ▪collagen synthesis	▪Complete epidermal regeneration ▪Continuing collagen synthesis

Source: Lultronics

Ablative laser skin resurfacing

The two most common lasers for skin resurfacing and wrinkle removal are carbon dioxide (CO_2) and Erbium:YAG lasers.

CO_2 laser appears to be somewhat more effective for treating deep wrinkles but has longer recovery time and tends to cause greater adverse reactions.

171

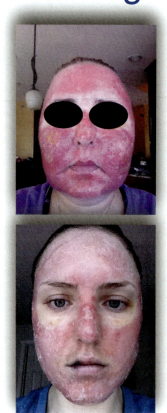

Ablative laser therapy for skin resurfacing

Some practitioners use both carbon dioxide and erbium:YAG lasers in a spontaneous procedure: erbium laser for fine lines and small wrinkles and carbon dioxide laser for deeper wrinkles.

Skin Resurfacing using Er:YAG 2940 Fractional

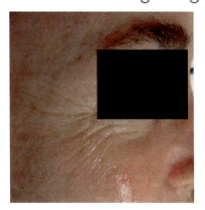
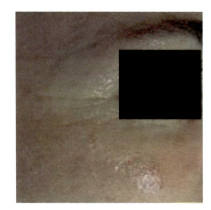

Before   After 3 sessions

172

Ablative laser skin resurfacing

Layers of the skin can be removed as superficial as Stratum Corneum or as deep as reticular dermis.

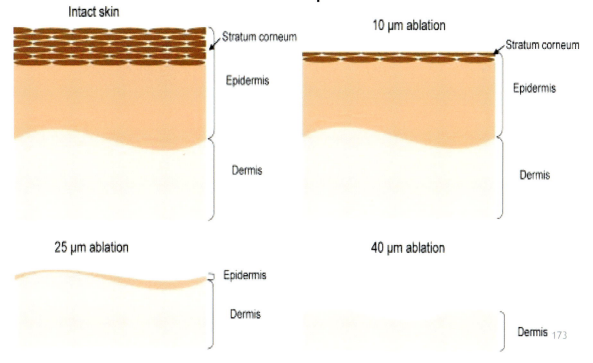

Procedures that you can perform with a Laser / IPL System

3 - Hyperpigmentation removal:

The most-commonly used lasers for the treatment of pigmented lesions, such as sun spots, age spots, and melasma are Pulsed Dye, Nd:YAG and fractional (Fraxel) lasers.

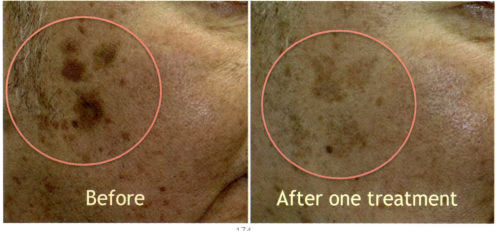

Mechanism of IPL Pigmentation Removal

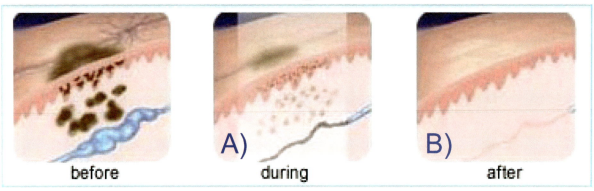

A) Unwanted skin pigments (melanin) are thoroughly fragmented without damage to the surrounding tissue.

B) Pigmented particles are then eliminated over weeks through a process which the fragmented pigments and damaged melanocytes to be absorbed by the body.

Mechanism of IPL Pigmentation Removal

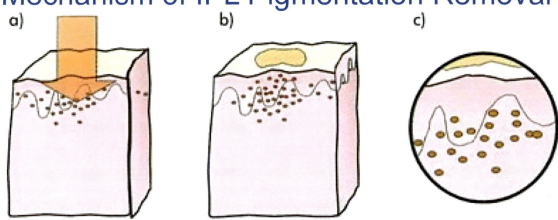

a) Areas of pigment absorb the light and are heated

b) The pigmented skin darkens initially and renews over the next 5 days

c) The excess pigment can continue to fade for several weeks afterwards.

Mechanism of IPL Pigmentation Removal

The pulses of light are absorbed by the excess melanin, creating heat that destroys the uppermost pigmented skin cells.

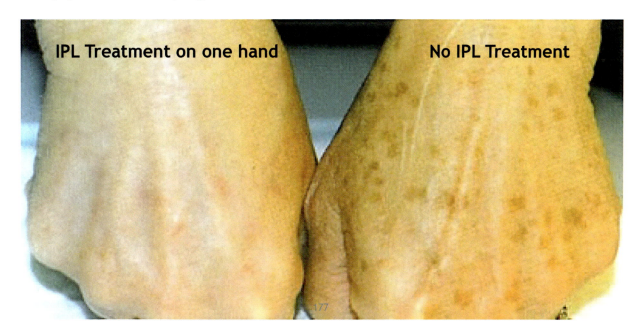

Mechanism of IPL Pigmentation Removal

1) Laser light is absorbed by the pigment melanin. The uppermost layer of the skin containing excess melanin in pigmentation lesions heats up and controllably burns. Then it scabs and slough off. The new skin grows without or with reduced pigmentation.

2) The molecular structure of pigment melanin will be fragmented and destroyed by laser thermal energy. Denatured melanin will no longer be recognized as domestic protein by immune cells and cleared up over the course of few days to weeks. The pigmentation lesions then will be absorbed and faded out gradually.

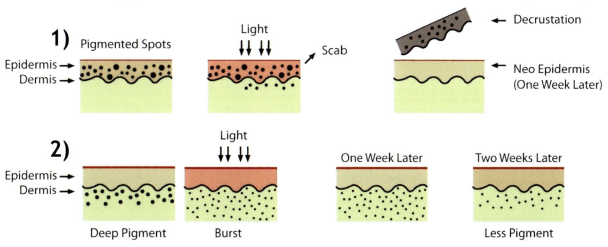

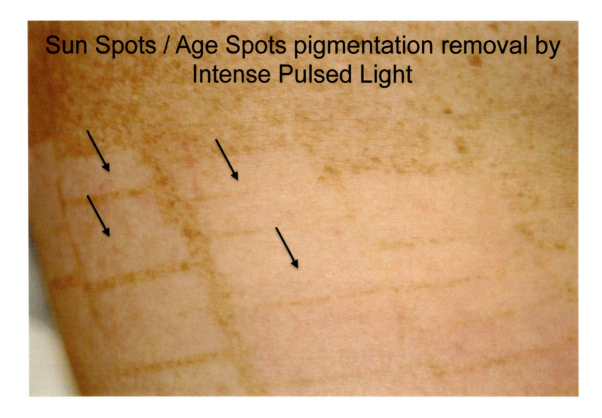

Sun Spots / Age Spots pigmentation removal by Intense Pulsed Light

179

Procedures that you can perform with a Laser / IPL System

4 - Vascular Lesion Removal

Vascular lesions include broken blood vessels on the face, unsightly veins on the legs, hemangiomas, spider nevi and certain birth marks such as port wine stains.

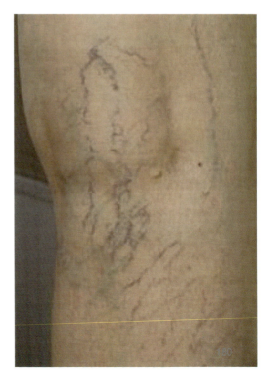

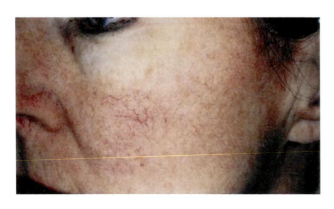

Mechanism of IPL Vascular Lesion Removal

A laser or IPL system precisely releases controlled strong pulses of photon energy that is absorbed by the superficial spider veins, and heating them up to a point where they are collapsed and / or destroyed, fragmented and eventually cleared by body immune cells.

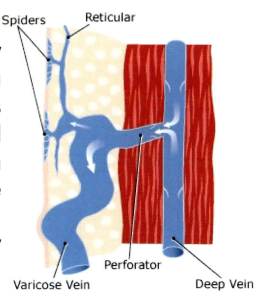

Suitable lasers for Vascular Lesion Removal

For reticular / spider vascular lesions, IPL is a common choice, as it is minimally invasive. Popular for treating these lesions are the pulsed dye, Nd:YAG and diode lasers.

For removal of larger varicose veins, injections of hypertonic solution (Sclerotherapy) is recommended.

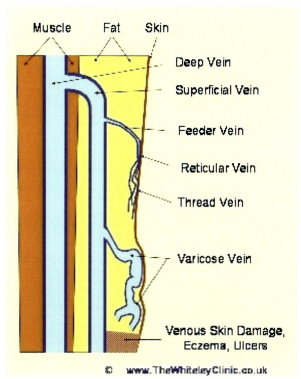

Mechanism of IPL Vascular Lesion Removal

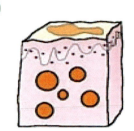 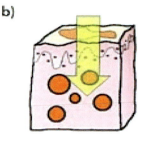 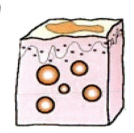

a)   b)   c)

a) Veins lying too close to the skin surface cause red lesions

b) The vessel absorbs the light and is heated

c) The vessel is destroyed and quickly clears.

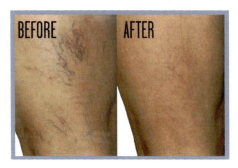 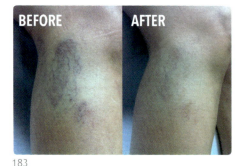

183

Mechanism of IPL Vascular Lesion Removal

Following treatment the vessels quickly clear and are re-absorbed by the body, leaving little or no trace of the original lesion.

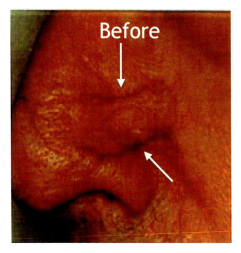 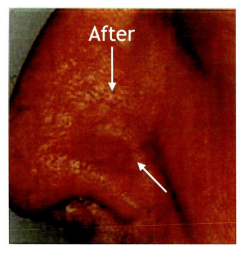

Before

After

184

Vein removal side effects

- Redness and a warm sensation are normal after the treatment.
- A cool pack may be applied to ease these symptoms.
- The vessels should fade quickly, and some disappear immediately.

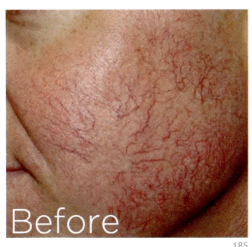 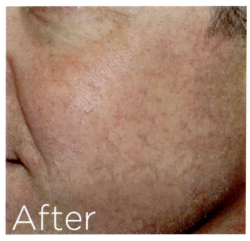

185

Procedures that you can perform with a Laser / IPL System

5 - Tattoo removal

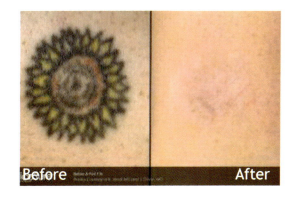

The Nd:YAG and CO2 lasers remain popular for tattoo removal, although some success can also be achieved with IPL.

Fragmented tattoo ink will be absorbed and cleared by body.

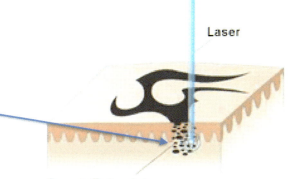

Target: Tattoo Inks

186

Laser / IPL Tattoo Removal

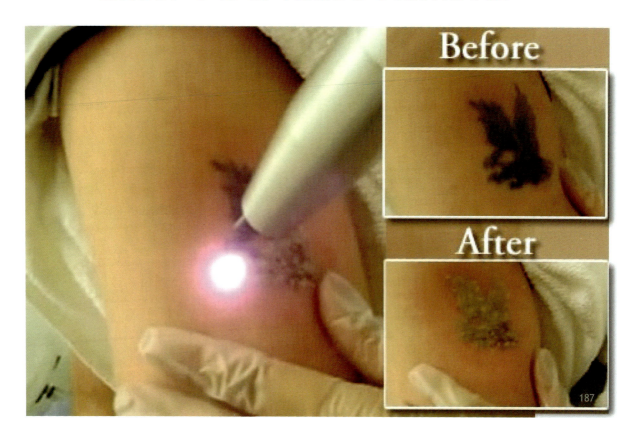

LASER TATTOO REMOVAL

While tattooing has been popular among a number of people, studies have shown that at least 50% of people with tattoos would like to remove them due to different reasons. Many individuals that appreciate tattoos and have many of them on their skin may become tired of the old ones and would consider removing them and perhaps acquiring new tattoos. Fortunately, laser tattoo removal is the safest and quickest treatment available with minimal side effects. Laser tattoo removal is the least of other more traditional methods of tattoo removal with some risk of scarring. Other treatment options for tattoo removal involve painful surgical excision and dermabrasion. However, they are rarely used today due to longer recovery, high possibility of developing scars and costs involved. 188

LASER TATTOO REMOVAL

Tattoo removal is a selective thermolysis procedure that delivers laser energy to the carbon particles or dyes that are found in skin tattoos, allowing selective destruction of the foreign pigment while minimizing damage to the surrounding skin. Lasers may be used on professional, amateur, cosmetic, medicinal, and traumatic tattoos. The different colors present in the tattoos may respond differently to laser tattoo removal. Tattoo removal by laser involves targeting the pigments by laser beam during multiple sessions. The pigment colors of the tattoo will break with a high-intensity laser beam. The light fragments the ink particles and the body absorbs these particles naturally. Tattoos generally require 3 - 8 treatments for complete removal.

189

Laser / IPL Tattoo Removal and ink color

Black, dark blue and brown tattoo ink are removed better and faster.

1064nm
TREATS
DARK INK

Orange, yellow and light green inks are more difficult to remove

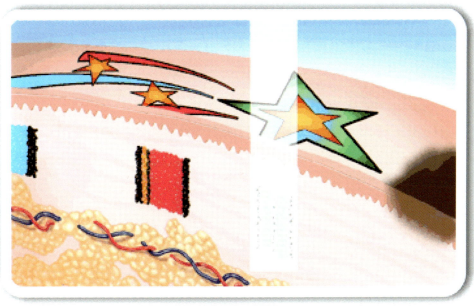

MECHANISM OF LASER TATTOO REMOVAL

However, the number of treatments varies with the individual and depends to many factors including size, color and depth of the tattoo, location and age. Several weeks is needed between sessions of laser treatment. After each session the tattoo becomes lighter. The color fades over a few weeks. Many patients tolerate the removal procedure without freezing the sensation. A topical anesthetic can be applied to alleviate any discomfort if required. Determining which tattoo ink is used, how deep or how much was used, helps to clear them as quickly as possible. Black tattoo pigment absorbs all laser wavelengths, making it the easiest to treat. Dark blue, dark green ink can be removed the best as well.

MECHANISM OF LASER TATTOO REMOVAL

Light red, light greens and yellows are the hardest to remove. The newer tattooing devices place the ink deeper and therefore the tattoo is harder to remove whereas, the older tattoos are easier to remove. Side effects of laser tattoo removal include redness, mild swelling or tenderness, crusting, a sunburn sensation, or itching right after laser treatment. Side effects may also manifest as hyperpigmentation, infection or pinpoint bleeding. Treated skin is sensitive and should be protected from sun exposure. It is recommended to apply an antibiotic ointment following the treatment and the wound should be covered with a protective dressing.

Disadvantages of Laser Tattoo Removal:

Expensive (can cost up to $5000).

Painful (sometimes more painful than applying the tattoo).

Risky (can damage and scar the skin).

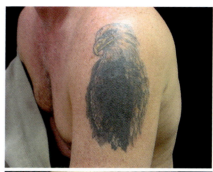

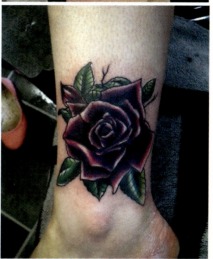

193

Alternative Tattoo Removal Methods

Dermabrasion (sanding the skin off until the tattoo is faded).

Salabrasion (rubbing the tattoo with a salt block until the tattoo is faded).

Excision (literally cutting out the tattoo and sewing the skin back together).

Skin Grafts (placing non-tattooed portions of the skin over the tattoo).

194

6 - Laser Hair Removal (LHR)

The success and safety of laser hair removal is highly dependent on the pigment present in both the skin and the hair of the patient being treated.

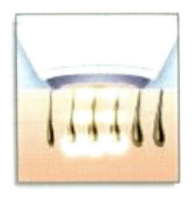 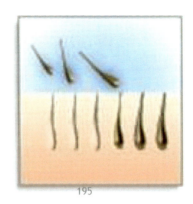 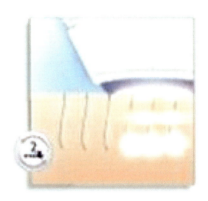

LASER HAIR REMOVAL

Hair removal lasers have been successfully used in cosmetic industry for several years providing satisfactory results. Lasers target terminal hairs with the pigment melanin thereby, the intense pulse of laser beam is absorbed primarily by the pigment in the hair follicle. Each light pulse lasts only for very small fraction of a second, so the energy from the beam is almost completely absorbed by the hair papilla without significant spreading to the surrounding tissue. Terminal hairs are thick, long, and usually pigmented with melanin. Hair on the scalp, underarms, genitals, and eyebrows chest, back, legs, and arms are examples of terminal hairs.

LASER HAIR REMOVAL

Short and non-pigmented hairs that can be found in most other areas of the body and face are called Vellus hairs. Age, ethnicity, weight, metabolism, medication, and hormones all play a role in the location, resilience, and thickness of hair. Lasers destroy hairs by targeting the bulge and papilla region. The light energy from the laser is converted to thermal energy in the hair follicle. This process is referred to selective photo thermolysis. It is selective because it targets only the hair and not the skin. Photo means light and thermolysis means destroying with heat. The bulge area of the hair follicle is involved in the hair cycling and regeneration while the papilla is the vascular structure of hair follicle and is associated with nutrition and oxygen supplementation.

LASER HAIR REMOVAL

Without normal follicle, hair cannot survive and falls off. In addition, lasers are most effective when target the hair follicle in its active phase of growth cycle called Anagen. Destroyed hairs are then either dissolved within the skin or rejected by the body within the next several days. A successful laser hair removal paradigm in achieved by repeated treatment since only a portion of all hairs in the body is in the Anagen phase at any given time. This varies in individuals and in different areas of the body usually from 20 to 85% of total hair. Some follicles are destroyed, while others are partially traumatized, reduced to fine hairs or subjected to extended quiescence.

LASER HAIR REMOVAL

Generally, about 30% of the hairs will not re-grow after a single treatment. It is difficult to predict how many treatments each individual will require to achieve the best long-term benefits. Therefore, multiple treatments are needed to provide the best results. FDA has approved laser treatment for permanent hair reduction and not permanent hair removal, which is endorsed by many cosmetic clinics. It is possible that with a sufficient number of treatments, true "permanent hair removal" can eventually be achieved. Taken together, after all the laser sessions have been completed, it takes approximately six months before one can make a final judgment regarding the success of the treatment.

Mechanism of IPL / Laser Hair Removal

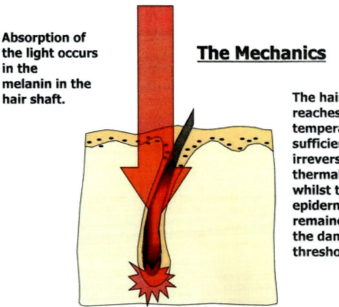

Absorption of the light occurs in the melanin in the hair shaft.

The Mechanics

The hair follicle reaches a temperature sufficient to cause irreversible thermal damage whilst the epidermis has remained below the damage threshold

Physicians administering laser or photo (light) therapy must first assess the patient's skin type to determine the appropriate dose – that is, the amount of exposure, which will provide beneficial effect whilst minimizing damage incurred. Similarly, researchers examining skin conditions need to cater their experimental design and treatments to individual variations in skin type.

Skin Type	Fitzpatrick Skin Type	Common Nationalities
1	Very fair- always burns in the sun and never tans	Celtic
2	Fair- burns in the sun and tans with great difficulty	Scandinavian
3	Fair- burns but tans gradually	Caucasian
4	Medium- Hardly ever burns and tans with ease	Mediterranean, Hispanic and some Asian
5	Light Brown- Rarely burns and tans profusely	Pakistani & Indian
6	Dark Brown- never burns in the sun and is deeply pigmented	African

The Fitzpatrick Classification Scale was developed in 1975 by dermatologist Thomas Fitzpatrick, MD. This scale classifies a person's complexion and their tolerance of sunlight. It is widely used by many practitioners to hair type for laser treatment, and to determine how someone will respond or react to facial treatments. Fitzpatrick skin type is governed by genetic factors and does not change throughout their lifetime, despite changes in facultative pigmentation (tanning).

CANDIDATES FOR LASER HAIR REDUCTION

People with coarse dark hair and light skin color respond the best to laser hair treatments. In clients with darker skin color that have more melanin in their skin, the skin tends to compete with the hair to absorb the light energy, resulting in potential damage to the skin. It is strongly recommended that to avoid tanning before any laser treatments. People with grey hair are the most difficult to treat as less energy is absorbed by the hair roots. All parts of the body can be treated with the exception of the area immediately surrounding the eyes. In women, the most common areas are underarms, bikini line, chin, upper lip, arms and legs.

EFFECTIVENESS OF LASER HAIR REDUCTION

In men the most common areas are the back, shoulders, chest and the beard area. Lasers can be used individually or in combinations for different skin and hair types to produce the best results. Treatments can be performed without anesthesia. There is some pain because the individual hair follicle is surrounded by nerve endings. While clients may be able to tolerate the procedure without the use of an anesthetic, others may find the application of an anesthetic cream helpful. However, in order to reduce the risk of thermal damage of the skin and scarring, it is highly recommended not to numb the area of treatment to have the client's feedback on the level of tolerance and optimal laser therapy.

203

For darker-skinned patients, the Nd:YAG and diode lasers are often the lasers of choice, and for lighter-skinned patients, IPL has proven effective.

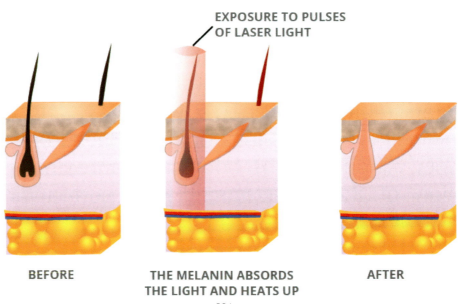

EXPOSURE TO PULSES OF LASER LIGHT

BEFORE

THE MELANIN ABSORDS THE LIGHT AND HEATS UP

AFTER

204

Mechanism of Laser / IPL Hair Removal + RF (RadioFrequency)

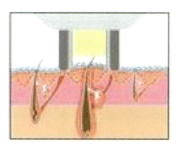

Fig. 1
Contact is made with skin and cooling begins.

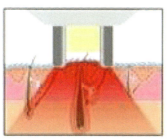

Fig. 2
Laser pre-heats target.

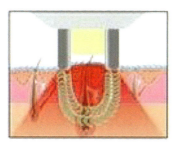

Fig. 3
RF is drawn toward heated target deep inside the dermis and both energies work to attack both the inside and outside of the target.

IPL Hair Reduction Steps

1. IPL uses a specially constructed xenon flash lamp and focusing optics.

2. The pulses of light are absorbed by melanin within the hairs, creating heat that destroys the hair root.

3. IPL destroys papilla and follicle to stop re-growth.

4. It removes unwanted hair through a process called selective photothermolysis.

EFFECTIVENESS OF LASER HAIR REDUCTION

Hair grows in cycles, so not every hair can be treated at the same time.

It's recommend that, during the first 3 months, treatment to be performed every 3 weeks.

After that, treatment should be carried on just once every month until the last treatment.

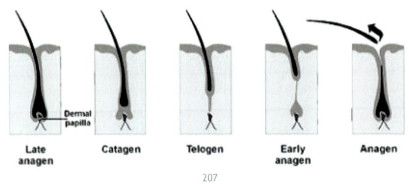

IPL / Laser Hair Removal and Hair Growth Cycle

Laser / IPL only is effective on hairs that are in active phase of hair growth stage , the "Anagen".

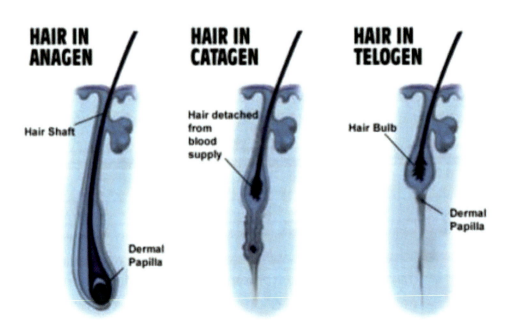

Thicker and darker hair follicles are located in deep dermis but easier to remove. They have much more melanin / chromophore that absorbs photon / thermal energy of the Laser. Conversely, superficial blond or grey hair are harder to destroy and are more persistent.

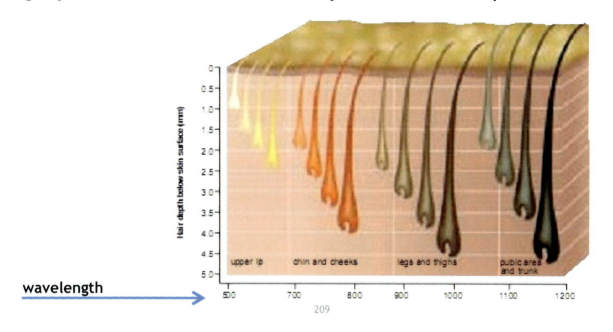

wavelength

ELECTROLYSIS vs LASER HAIR REMOVAL

Electrolysis treats one hair at a time by inserting a fine probe into what is hopefully the base of the hair and destroys the hair root using small electric shocks. Unlike electrolysis laser uses a wide beam, which treats many hairs at once. However, electrolysis is useful in removing hairs from small areas such as the area around the eyes and in the nose. Laser hair removal is not only faster than electrolysis but can treat hairs that are untreatable by electrolysis. The laser offers a permanent reduction in both the amount of hair and also often a reduction in thickness and color of hairs that may grow back.

IPL / Laser Hair Removal Face & under arms

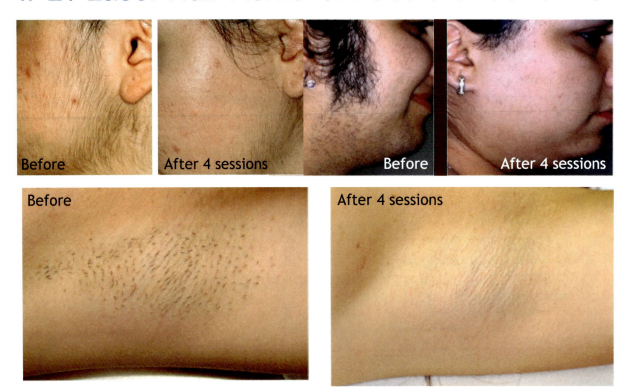

Before | After 4 sessions | Before | After 4 sessions

Before | After 4 sessions

211

EFFECTIVENESS OF LASER HAIR REDUCTION

Long-term studies have indicated that all the hairs that respond to the laser are permanently destroyed thus laser is considered the treatment of choice for those who desire to reduce their unwanted hair for a long period of time. In certain circumstances, there maybe persistent hairs that take several treatments before they are destroyed. A realistic expectation is an 80-90% hair reduction. Often, any remaining hairs are finer and lighter than previously. At least two weeks prior to laser hair reduction treatment waxing, plucking, threading, electrolysis and bleaching should be avoided. Makeup can absorb laser energy and interfere its effect; therefore, it is important not to wear make up when facial laser procedure is performed.

Most wanted areas for Laser Hair Removal and Average Price Range per session

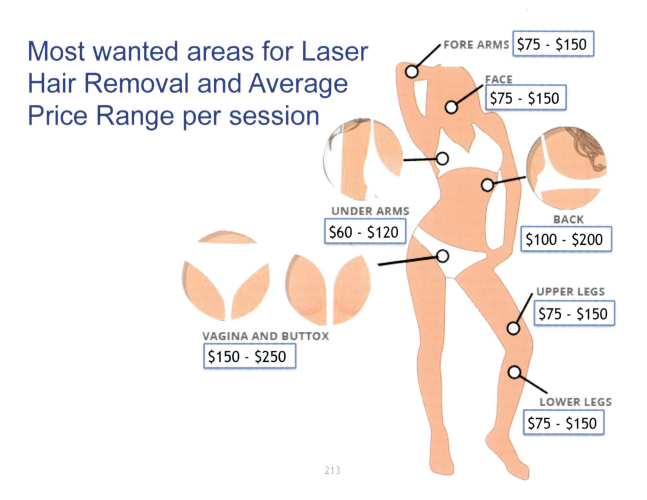

FORE ARMS $75 - $150

FACE $75 - $150

UNDER ARMS $60 - $120

BACK $100 - $200

UPPER LEGS $75 - $150

LOWER LEGS $75 - $150

VAGINA AND BUTTOX $150 - $250

213

Procedures that you can perform with a Laser / IPL System
7 - Acne Treatment by Laser / IPL

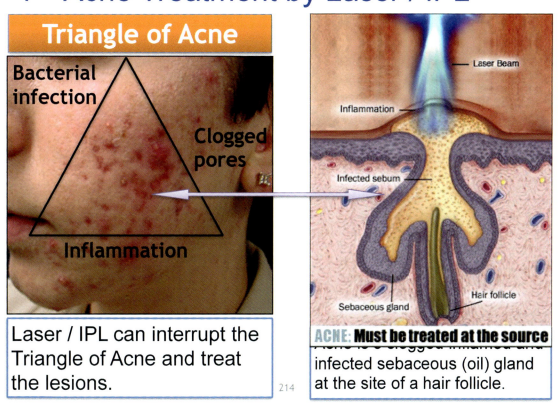

Triangle of Acne

Bacterial infection

Clogged pores

Inflammation

Laser / IPL can interrupt the Triangle of Acne and treat the lesions.

Laser Beam

Inflammation

Infected sebum

Sebaceous gland

Hair follicle

ACNE: **Must be treated at the source**

infected sebaceous (oil) gland at the site of a hair follicle.

214

Mechanism of IPL / Laser Acne Removal

A high energy pulse of light is applied to the treatment area.

The intense light is absorbed by the targeted subcutaneous oil glands damaging and permanently disabling them while destroying the bacteria that breed inside the glands.

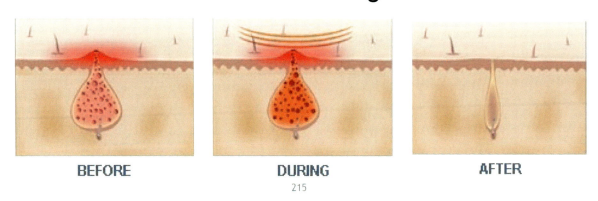

BEFORE   DURING   AFTER

215

Suitable systems for Laser Acne and Acne Scars Removal

For deeper acne scars, the CO2 laser remains the treatment of choice.

Erbium:YAG, fractional laser and IPL have shown considerable success on more superficial acnes and acne scarring.

Alternatively, for the treatment of active acne, Blue / Green LED and Argon Electrode High-frequency technology has proven to be quite effective.

216

IPL and Acne treatment, Before and After

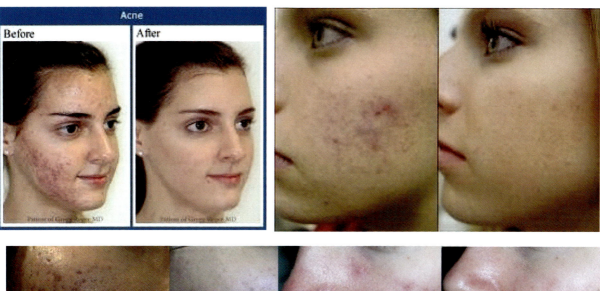

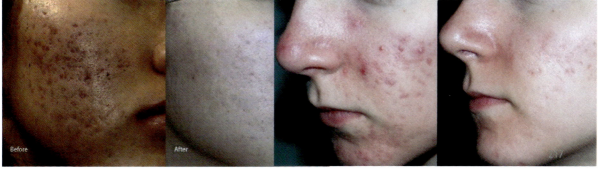

LASER LIPOLYSIS (LYPOLASER)

Lipolaser has been approved by FDA and as a non-invasive, painless laser treatment for spot fat reduction and aesthetic body contouring. The Lipolaser's treatment is considered one of the most effective methods to reduce the appearance of cellulite and improve body contour. The Lipolaser targets fat tissue layers in any areas of the body including waistlines, arms, legs, thighs, buttocks and back. Lipolaser is a non-surgical adipose treatment, which reduces accumulated fat in fat cells called adipocytes (such as cellulite). It brings the broken down fat to the muscular layer where blood capillary flow is well distributed. Broken fat then is absorbed in the blood stream and naturally excreted.

Combining a healthy diet and regular exercise provide best results after a Lipolaser procedure. At the cellular level, during treatments, the fat cells become permeable by laser. When the laser radiates fat cells or adipocytes the contents of the cells move out of the cell membrane and become liquefied and are easily removed from the blood. The breakdown of fat cells is known as lipolysis, a process that converts fat to free fatty acids, water and glycerol, which in turn are further processed through the body's natural metabolic functions.

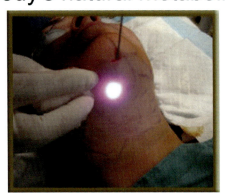 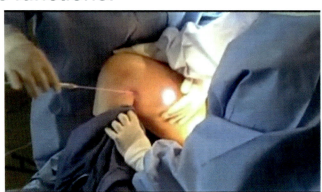

Preparation of clients prior to a Laser / IPL treatment

- Assessment
- Suitability
- Consultation
- Preparation
- Medical History
- Consent forms

Client suitability and education:

- Assess the clients' skin type, hair colour, thickness and location of hair, presence of a tan, previous hair removal methods, medical history (ovarian or thyroid disease, diabetes, medications, history of abnormal scarring, history of cold sore outbreaks in the treatment area, or past isotretinoin use), and presence of tattoos or moles in the treatment area.

- Discuss realistic outcomes (need for multiple treatment sessions, potential need for maintenance sessions, and the possibility of variable responses to treatment)

- Provide pre-treatment instructions (no tanning, plucking, waxing, electrolysis, etc.) Assess whether there is a need for prophylactic antiviral medication.

- Perform a patch test prior to full treatment.

Documentation & Records

Owners need to keep records and have them available on site, including:

- Laser operators authorized on the laser(s) found on-site

- Laser operator(s) qualifications, education, test results and safety training

- Standard operating procedures (SOP)

Safety checklist:

- Setup of laser controlled area with signs, window barriers, etc.

- Confirmation of eyewear type and availability

- Patient protection, including removal or covering of reflective surfaces (e.g. jewellery)

- Safety equipment such as smoke evacuator, fire safety & equipment.

Assessment of the skin color and type

In order to ascertain the most appropriate device setting to use, first an assessment of the client's skin type according to Fitzpatrick scale is necessary. This system is based on a person's response to sun exposure in terms of the degree of burning and tanning the individual experience. Below is the summary of Fitzpatrick classification:

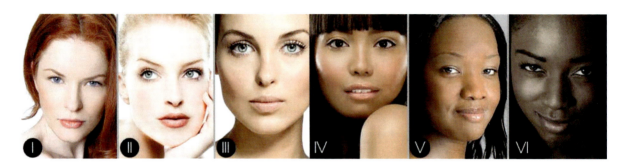

223

TYPE 1: Highly sensitive, always burns, never tans. Example: Red hair with freckles.

TYPE 2: Very sun sensitive, burns easily, tans minimally. Example: Fair-skinned, fair-haired Caucasians.

TYPE 3: Sun sensitive skin, sometimes burns, slowly tans to light brown. Example: Darker Caucasians, European mix.

TYPE 4: Minimally sun sensitive, burns minimally, always tans to moderate brown. Example: Mediterranean, European, Asian, Hispanic, American Indian.

TYPE 5: Sun-insensitive skin, rarely burns, tans well. Example: Hispanics, Afro-American, Middle Eastern.

TYPE 6: Sun-insensitive, never burns, deeply pigmented. Example: Afro-American, African, Middle Eastern.

224

- The effectiveness of laser / IPL treatment is highly dependent on patient cooperation.

- There are many things a patient can inadvertently do to decrease either the safety or effectiveness of their treatment.

- It is, therefore, imperative to follow directions and instructions by the practitioner.

225

Preparation prior to Laser / IPL treatment

- No make-up must be worn before the treatment. It may interfere with the laser radiation and either result in skin burn or ineffective treatment.

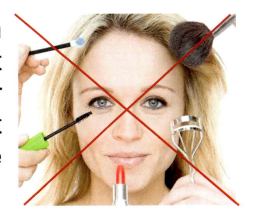

- No creams, lotions, foundations, sun blocks, tanning sprays at the time of treatment.

- Jewellers, neckless, rings and earnings must be taken off during the treatment to eliminate the risk of accidental reflection.

226

Lotions, creams, makeup, and deodorant must be removed before treatment because they can obstruct or refract laser light negatively.

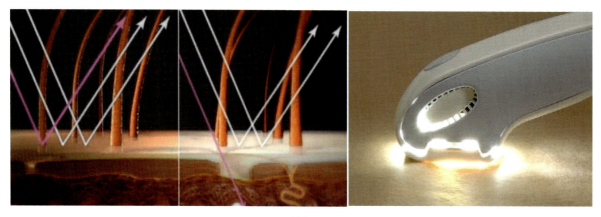

227

Preparation prior to Laser / IPL treatment

The hair needs to be in the follicle at the time of treatment and lasers target the pigment melanin in the hair beneath the surface of the skin.

Because of this, patients should not wax, tweeze, bleach, thread, or use depilatory agents for 4 weeks prior to treatment.

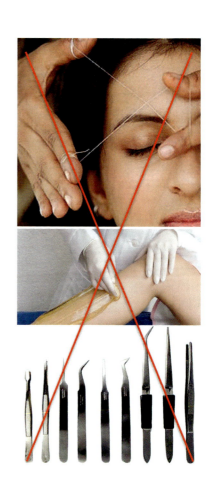

228

Preparation prior to Laser / IPL treatment

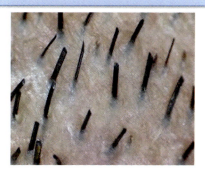

- For Laser hair removal, shaving or clipping can be done. These methods allow the hair to stay in the follicle.

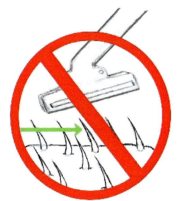

- It is usually advisable to see some hair growth on the day of treatment. Shaving the area must be done 2-3 days prior to the appointment.

- Shaving must be performed with the hair growth direction not against.

229

Preparation prior to Laser / IPL treatment

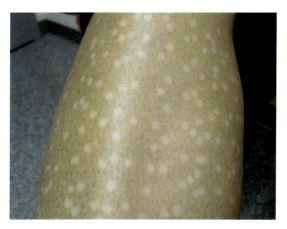

Tanned skin, either sun- or spray-tanned must not be treated with laser / IPL. Treating skin with a tan can produce white "striping" which can take several months to fade.

Tanning is the single most important act that patients do to decrease the effectiveness of their treatment. Tanning should be avoided for 4-6 weeks prior to treatment if lasers is to be used.

Preparation prior to Laser / IPL treatment

During the course of treatment in case of exposure to sun, sunscreen with a SPF of at least 30 must be applied as a thick layer 20 min is recommended.

Self-tanning creams and sprays need to completely fade out before laser treatment.

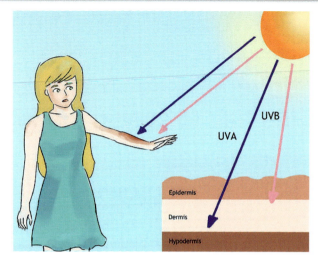

Wide spectrum Sun block lotion prevents penetration of both UVA and UVB into the skin.

231

Preparation prior to Laser / IPL treatment

- Use of all Vitamin A-type creams, Glycolic acid products and toners a week before treatment because the may lead to thin thinner more delicate skin.

- These product increases the skin fragility sensitivity and makes it prone to thermal damage.

- No plans for any major events for 2 to 3 days after the fist IPL treatment.

- It is not recommended to take hot bath, sauna and have intense physical work out immediately after laser treatment.

232

Laser / IPL Contraindications

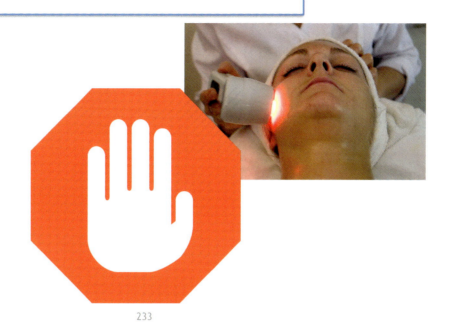

233

Laser: Contraindications

While laser treatments are safe and effective for most women and men, there are some people who will not be good candidates for these types of treatments.

Here is a general contraindication list that should be considered by anyone who is thinking of undergoing any laser or light based treatments:

- Sun exposure and/or artificial tanning
- Pregnancy
- Internal defibrillator or pacemaker
- Cancer
- Epilepsy
- Diabetes
- Active Herpes Simplex in the treatment area
- Vitiligo (hypo-pigmentation) or hyper-pigmentation
- Lupus
- Porphyria

234

Laser / IPL Contraindications

Sun exposure and/or artificial tanning during the last four (4) weeks for skin type I/II/III and 8 weeks for skin type IV/V is not recommended.

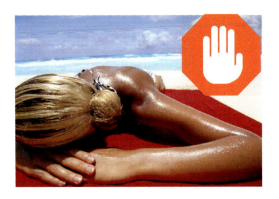

Anyone who is considering undergoing any laser treatments, must make sure wearing a titanium dioxide/zinc oxide SPF 30+ every day.

Laser / IPL Contraindications

Pregnancy - Pregnant women or nursing are advised from receiving any laser treatments. To date there have been no studies conducted to see what effects laser treatments may have on the unborn child.

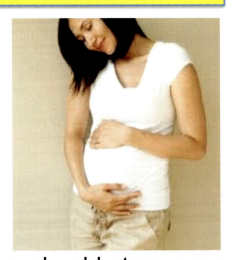

en should stay away from any type of cosmetic/elective procedures. In terms of hair reduction the hormones of women who are pregnant or nursing are unstable and will cause hair reduction treatments to be less effective.

Never perform Laser in these conditions:

Cancer - Skin cancer patients should not undergo any laser treatment.

Epilepsy - Light based treatment may trigger an epileptic attack.

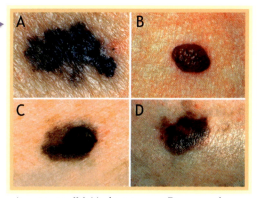

A: stage IV Melanoma, B: a mole, C and D: stage II and III Melanoma.

Diabetes – Unstable diabetes patients should never be treated as they will have problems with healing. Any laser treatment on stable diabetes patients need to be executed in close collaboration with the patient's physician.

237

No Laser treatment in higly sensetive Skin

Accutane or any related acne medication: No Accutane, oral Isotretinoin-Roaccutane, Tretinoin-Retin A (or any related drug) for a minimum of 6 months prior to undergoing any laser treatment.

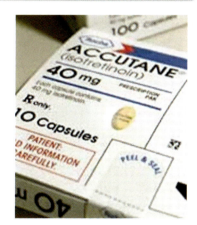

Active Herpes Simplex: No laser treatment on cold sore infection. Treatment is possible once the outbreak is healed.

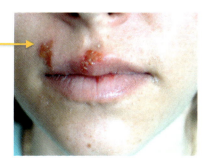

238

Laser / IPL Contraindications

Vitiligo (hypo-pigmentation) or hyper-pigmentation: individuals with these conditions should not be treated with laser at all. They may develop more discolouration.

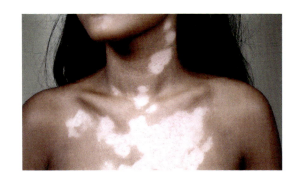

Any active inflammatory skin condition: e.g. No laser treatment on eczema, psoriasis, infection, rash or any type of dermatitis at the treatment site (because it may aggravate the condition).

239

Laser / IPL Contraindications

Lupus: is a chronic inflammatory disease that occurs when the body's immune system attacks ones own tissues and organs. Light Therapy may aggravate the skin condition.

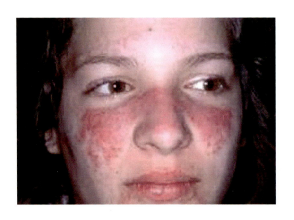

In a tendency to develop Hyperpigmentation after any laser or light therapy the treatment should be stopped.

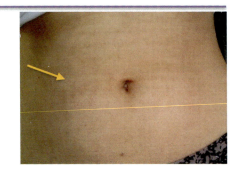

240

Laser / IPL Contraindications

No laser / IPL in people with a tendency of **Keloid Scar** formation after wound healing.

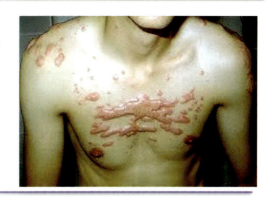

Porphyria: (A blood disorder that makes sensitive to light). Extreme sensitivity or allergy to light.

241

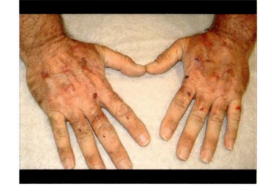

Laser / IPL Contraindications

No Laser / IPL treatment in dark skin color (South Asian, African) / A dark tan.

The major risk of laser treatment in darker skin is that the skin can burn and become hyper or worse hypopigmented with loss of skin color.

242

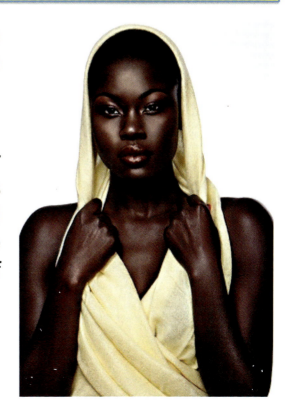

Side effects of the laser treatment process may include:

- pain

- bruising and swelling

- redness and inflammation

- blistering

- herpes simplex outbreaks and bacterial infections

- temporary skin lightening or darkening

- darkening/lightening of tattoos

- freckle loss or lightening of moles

- permanent skin pigment changes or scarring (rare)

- exacerbation of pre-existing skin conditions

- allergic reactions to anaesthetic creams

243

Cosmetic Laser / IPL
post-treatment

Cosmetic Laser / IPL post-treatment

- If facial area is being treated, after and between the laser treatment sessions sunscreen (with at least SPF* 30) must be used to protect the skin.

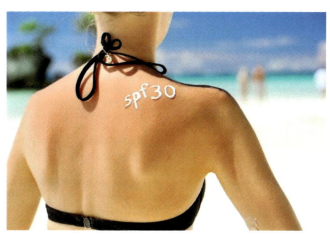

*Sun Protection Factor

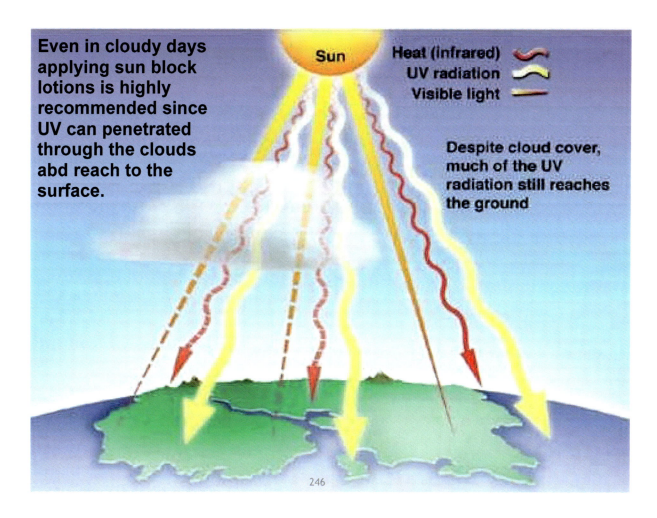

Even in cloudy days applying sun block lotions is highly recommended since UV can penetrated through the clouds abd reach to the surface.

Sun

Heat (infrared)
UV radiation
Visible light

Despite cloud cover, much of the UV radiation still reaches the ground

Cosmetic Laser / IPL post-treatment

- After laser / IPL treatment wash treated areas gently with a mild cleanser.
- If the treated area is irritated, no rubbing with a towel – rather pat dry.

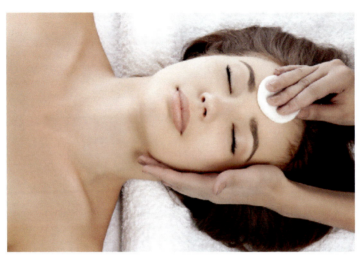

247

Cosmetic Laser / IPL post-treatment

- In order to prevent scarring, do not rub, scratch, or pick at the treated area while red discolouration present after a laser / IPL treatment.
- Avoid rubbing or pressure caused by clothing on the treated area.

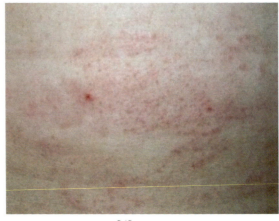

248

Cosmetic Laser / IPL post-treatment

- Resume Retinol (Vitamin A) and Retin "A" products one week post-treatment.

H3C, CH3 — CH2OH
Retinol
CH3

H3C, CH3 — H / C=O
Retinal (retinaldehyde)
CH3

H3C, CH3 — COOH
Retinoic Acid
CH3

H3C, CH3 H3C
β-carotene
CH3 H3C CH3

RETINOL
Vitamin Enriched
Day Cream with SPF 20 Sunscreen

Cosmetic Laser / IPL post-treatment

- Apply moisturizers and / or Vitamin E to the area for re-hydration.

- If crusting develops few days after the treatment, it should be allowed to fall off (slough off) naturally. Do not pick or scratch crust.

- Resume normal skin care regimens (i.e. make-up, moisturizers, deodorant, or shaving after treatment if there is no blistering or crusting.

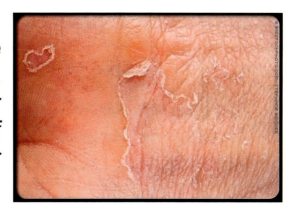

Cosmetic Laser / IPL post-treatment

- Use skin care products that are free from alcohol, dyes, and perfumes for one week post-treatment.

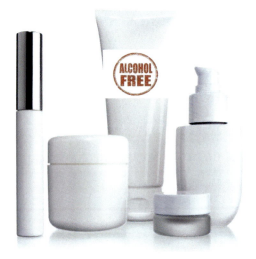

251

Cosmetic Laser / IPL post-treatment

- If there is any break or blistering of the skin, an antibiotic ointment should be used such as Polysporin.

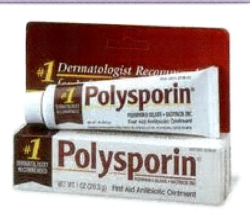

- If there are any signs of infection such as redness, tenderness, or pus, the client must contact the office.

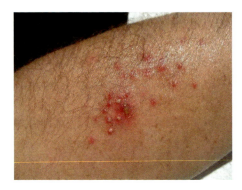

252

Cosmetic Laser / IPL post-treatment

- Activities such as swimming and use of hot tubs should be avoided for the first 2 - 3 days or until any redness, crusting, or blisters have resolved.

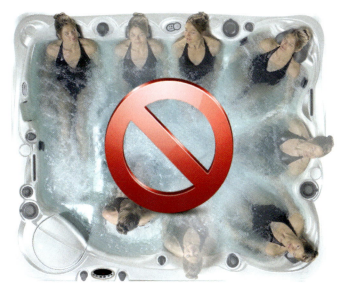

253

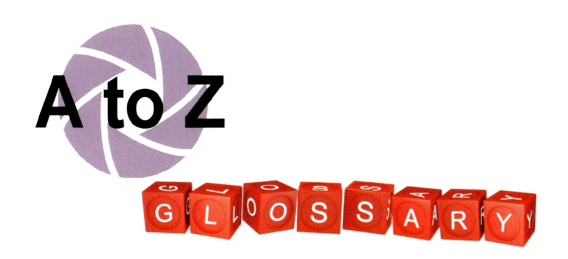

254

ANSI: the American National Standards Institute - a private, non-profit organization that administers the US voluntary standardization and conformity assessment system.

Authorized personnel: Individuals approved by management (business owner) to operate, maintain, service or install laser equipment.

Baseline eye examination: an eye examination that used to establish a basis for comparison in the event of an accidental laser injury.

Beam: the pulsed or continuous output from a laser.

Cataract: clouding of the lens of the eye.

Coherent: a beam of light characterized by a fixed phase relationship or single wavelength (i.e. monochromatic).

Danger: indicates an imminently hazardous situation which, if not avoided, will result in death or serious injury e.g. retinal burn from direct exposure to the laser beam

Diffuse reflection: change of the spatial distribution of a beam of radiation when it is reflected from a rough surface in many directions

Direct beam: the output beam from the laser, prior to any reflection or absorption.

Electromagnetic radiation: the flow of energy at the speed of light in the form of electric and magnetic fields. Gamma rays, X-ray, ultraviolet, visible, infrared, and radio waves occupy various portions of the electromagnetic spectrum and differ only in frequency, wavelength and photon energy. **Incidental personnel**: those whose work makes it possible (but unlikely) that they will be exposed to laser energy sufficient to damage their eyes or skin (i.e. clerical or supervisory personnel who do not work directly with lasers).

Infrared radiation (IR): invisible radiation wavelengths from about 700 nm to 1,000,000 nm (1 millimetre). Hair removal lasers operate between 700 and 1400 nm.

Irradiance: the radiant power incident per unit area upon a surface, expressed in W/cm2 (Symbol: E). **Joule (J)**: the unit used to measure the energy of a laser pulse.

kW/cm2: a kilowatt per square centimetre [see Watt].

Laser: acronym for **L**ight **A**mplification by **S**timulated **E**mission of **R**adiation.

Laser controlled area: an area that is appropriately enclosed so that no laser radiation above the maximum permissible exposure inadvertently escapes to injure unsuspecting persons. This area is subject to the control and supervision of the laser safety officer and must contain the nominal hazard zone (NHZ) unless special safety features are incorporated into the room.

Laser personnel: those who work routinely in the laser environment and are normally fully protected by engineering controls and/or administrative procedures (i.e. operators or service providers).

Laser safety officer (LSO): a person who is authorized by management (business owner) to be responsible for the laser safety program in the facility. The LSO is responsible for monitoring and overseeing the control of laser hazards.

Light: electromagnetic radiation having wavelengths between approximately 400 to 700 nm and which are perceptible to human vision (aka "visible light").

Melanin: a group of naturally occurring dark pigments found in skin and hair which absorb infrared laser radiation.

Maximum Permissible Exposure (MPE): the level of laser radiation to which an unprotected person may be exposed without adverse biological changes in the eye or skin i.e. injury

Nanometers (nm): a unit of length equal to one thousand millionth of a meter (10^{-9} m) and used in the measure of wavelengths of optical radiation i.e. ultraviolet, visible and infrared radiation.

Nd:YAG: notation for one of the lasing media in some lasers which produces the infrared radiation i.e. neodymium:yttrium-aluminum-garnet.

Nominal Hazard Zone (NHZ): the space within which the level of the direct, reflected, or scattered radiation during normal operation exceeds the applicable maximum permissible exposure. This zone is usually smaller than and within the laser controlled area.**Optical density (OD)**: a material's ability to absorb laser radiation, as used in protective eyewear. **OD number**: a measure of the safety of protective eyewear by how much the laser radiation is

reduced when it passes through the protective eyewear (see page 15) **Radiation**: Emission and propagation of energy in the form of particles or waves.

Retina: The delicate multilayered light-sensitive membrane lining the inner posterior chamber of the eyeball that contains the rods and cones, and is connected by the optic nerve to the brain.

Specular reflection: change of the spatial distribution of a beam of radiation when it is reflected from a mirror-like surface in one direction

Visible light: electromagnetic radiation having wavelengths between approximately 400 and 700 nm and which are perceptible to human vision (aka "light").**Wavelength**: The distance between one peak or crest of a wave of light or other electromagnetic radiation and the next corresponding peak or crest.

Watt/cm2: a watt per square centimetre.

Watt (W): a unit of power equal to one joule per second.

The End